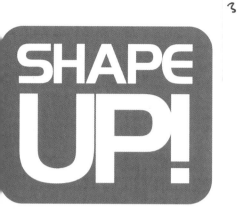

TAILOR-MADE TRAINING FOR
MALE BODY
TYPES

JOHN SHEPHERD

A & C BLACK • LONDON

First published in 2008
A & C Black Publishers Ltd
38 Soho Square
London W1D 3HB
www.acblack.com

Copyright © John Shepherd

ISBN 978 1 4081 0047 9

A CIP catalogue record for this book is available from the British Library.

Acknowledgements
Cover image © Grant Pritchard
Inside photography © Grant Pritchard, except pp. 4, 70 Bananastock; 124 Comstock; 142 (r) Corbis; 23, 31 Istock; 61 John Shepherd; 60, 104, 105, 108, 111, 113, 117, 122, 123, 137, 138 (l+r), 139, 145, 146 Punchstock; v, 27, 67, 71, 75, 87, 90, 115, 127, 128, 130, 131, 132, 133, 141, 142 (l), 149 (l+r) Shutterstock.
Designed by James Watson
Illustration © p. 3 Jeff Edwards
Thanks to Patrick Dale, James Conaghan and Jacqui Ball of Solar Fitness, Cyprus, for modelling and assisting with the organisation of the photo shoot. Solar Fitness runs personal trainer and fitness instructor courses on the island – for further information see www.solarfitness.com.

Note
Whilst every effort has been made to ensure the content of this book is as technically accurate as possible, neither the author nor the publishers can accept responsibility for any injury or loss sustained as a result of the use of this material.

This book is produced using paper that is made from wood grown in managed, sustainable forests. It is natural, renewable and recyclable. The logging and manufacturing processes conform to the environmental regulations of the country of origin.

Typeset in URWGrotesk by Palimpsest Book Production Limited, Grangemouth, Stirlingshire.

Printed and bound in China by South China Printing Co.

CONTENTS

ACKNOWLEDGEMENTS

In writing this book I became personally aware of just how much fitness can help you through life. I've trained regularly for over 25 years, and have sometimes taken for granted (or even not realised!) the holistic and wellbeing benefits of working out. In life you never know what's around the corner, but if you are fit and feeling good about yourself you'll be in the best position to challenge and deal with whatever lurks just out of sight.

I would specifically like to thank Grant Pritchard for taking the majority of the photographs in this book, and the guys at Solar Fitness Qualification in Cyprus – Pat, Jim, Jacqui and Vicky – for modelling and generally helping out. Also, Caroline Sandry for collaborating with me to write the women's version of this book. Thanks also to all at A&C Black Publishers for developing these projects and knocking them into shape.

www.johnshepherdfitness.co.uk

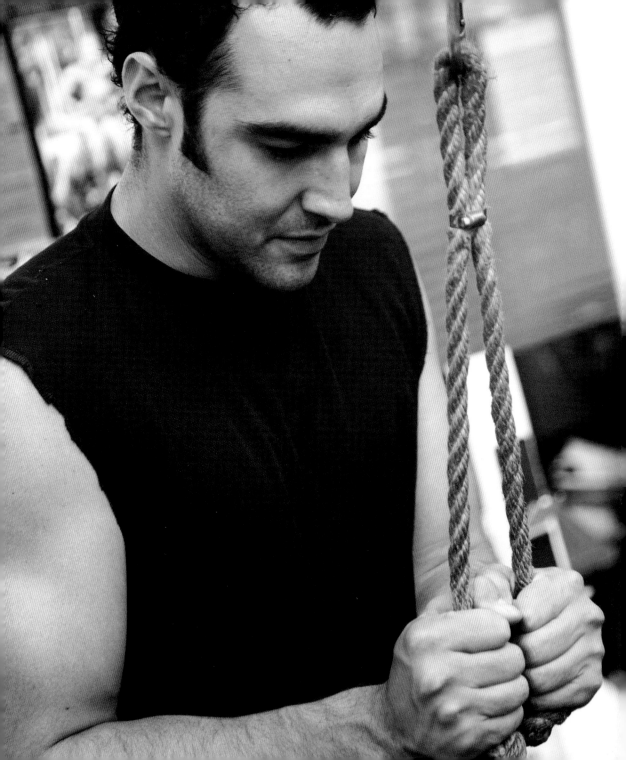

INTRODUCTION

A few years ago I interviewed Dave Prowse. Prowse is best known for playing Darth Vader in the *Star Wars* films (iv, v and vi), but he was also one of Britain's leading bodybuilders. The first thing he said to me after shaking hands was 'You're a "mesomorphic-ectomorph".' I was a little taken aback at this quick, but astute, guide to my body type. In laymen's terms, Prowse was explaining that I was muscled, well-proportioned but slim! I was a little upset at this as I thought I was more endo-mesomorphic (bigger) than Prowse thought I was!

As men, we are becoming increasingly concerned about our appearance – probably more so than at any other time in history. Media images of 'six packs' abound, and if we're carrying a 'little too much' around the middle we can feel under pressure and negative about ourselves. And to this I must also add the perhaps even more serious pressure placed on us by the current 'obesity epidemic'. In short, many of us need to lose weight to enjoy a healthier and longer life. I've written this book with this goal – and many others, such as building muscle – in mind. I aim to provide you with information, advice and training plans that will work. This means getting the most from your body type. Your physiology will influence how you shape up, but understanding this will enable you to get maximum returns from your training and your diet.

In this book you'll find sections on resistance and CV training and training planning, for example. Each explains what exercises and programmes work best for *your* body type and not some idealised standard. I present realistic expectations. With constant references to nutrition and supplements (as well as specific sections on these subjects), you'll discover all the information you need to achieve safely, quickly and effectively 'your best body', whatever your age, fitness or sports goals.

John Shepherd

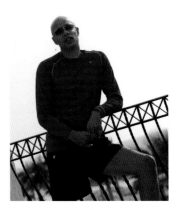

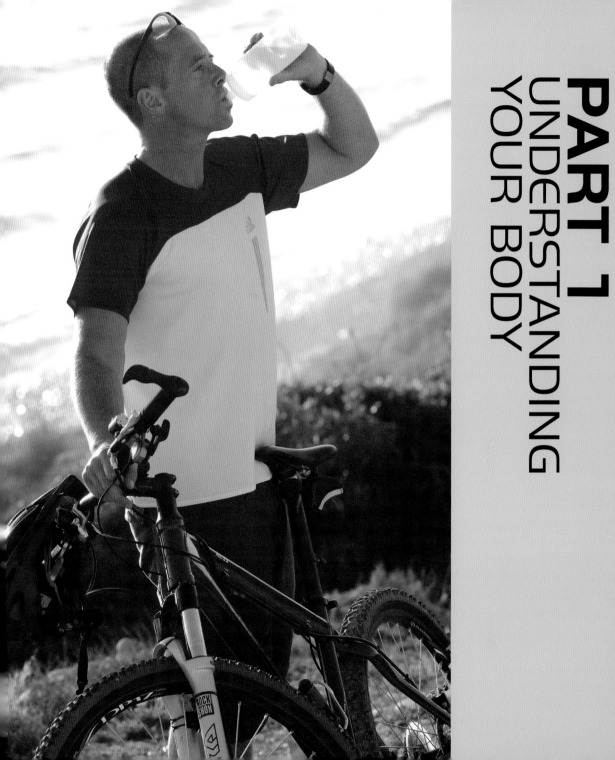

PART 1
UNDERSTANDING YOUR BODY

1

UNDERSTANDING YOUR BODY AND KNOWING YOUR BODY TYPE

We're not all the same, are we? Sounds obvious, but how many times do you pick up a workout/men's lifestyle magazine and see a guy on the cover, or doing a workout, who could have been sculpted by Michelangelo? The Adonis – or, as I'll indicate, 'true' mesomorph – is more the exception than the norm. These guys have inherited a body type – with narrow waists, broad shoulders, puffed chest and long limbs – that will gain muscle, but crucially look 'right' when carrying it. Many other guys don't have this body type; they may be slim and wiry (ectomorphs) or larger and rounder (endomorphs). However, whatever our body type, we can maximise our shape, strength, power and heart and lung capacity (cardiovascular (CV) fitness) throughout our lives. We just need to know how – and this is where the information in this book comes in.

I must explain that no body type is inherently better at the outset than any other. Each has its own abilities, strengths and weaknesses. Whichever type we possess (or we may have an amalgamation of the three) can be conditioned to respond positively to our training and lifestyle goals by following the right programme.

This part of the book will provide you with the information needed to identify your body type (and current body shape). It will also give you an overview of the key aspects of male physiology. Getting a grasp on all this will make it much easier to relate to and use the information provided in the practical training sections later in the book. As an example, knowing what type of fibres your muscles are made from will provide you with a much greater understanding of the ways you can train them via different weight training systems – for example, to gain muscle size, power and definition. I also provide some health-related information – notably on body weight, fat levels and obesity. These are presented to indicate just why embarking on a fitness programme that reflects your body type could be the most important thing you've ever done for yourself.

What's your body type?

As I've indicated, there are three main body types (or, more specifically, 'somatotypes') – these are ectomorphs, mesomorphs and endomorphs. This basic classification owes much to the work of the psychologist William Sheldon in the mid-twentieth century. In laymen's terms, these types can be described as 'thin', 'athletic' and 'fat'. Sheldon believed that each had distinct physiological (and psychological) traits. Although his work is perhaps over-stated, it provides a highly valuable starting point for the analysis of male (and female) body types. This is because it is possible to identify the ways that these types will typically respond physiologically to training. I must also point out that as Dave 'Darth Vader' Prowse said to me (see Introduction), most of us are actually an amalgamation of the three body types. I'm an 'ectomorph/mesmorph' – meaning slimmer, athletic and relatively muscled, rather than big, athletic and well-muscled, an 'endomorph-mesomorph'. In fact, Sheldon identified 'seven parts', 1–7 for each somatotype – with 1 being the minimum and 7 the maximum number of parts attributable to that somatotype. This is known as 'dominant somatotype'. For example, 2–6–3 indicates low endomorphy—high mesomorphy—low ectomorphy (note variations to this system exist which identify parts to decimal points).

To simplify things I have provided five somatotypes, one of which should be close to yours. Throughout the book I make reference to these in terms of relevant training options and nutrition.

Note: You should also refer to the information provided in Table 1 when determining your body type, and note too the difference between body shape and body type (see page 7). You should also use the Body Mass Index table on page 10 to identify whether you are underweight, of ideal weight or overweight.

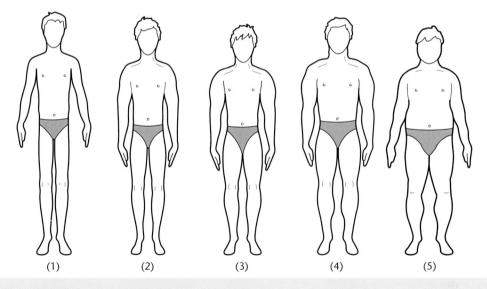

(1)   (2)   (3)   (4)   (5)

Fig. 1.1: *The five main body types: (1) Ectomorph (2) Ecto-mesomorph (3) Mesomorph (4) Meso-endomorph (5) Endomorph*

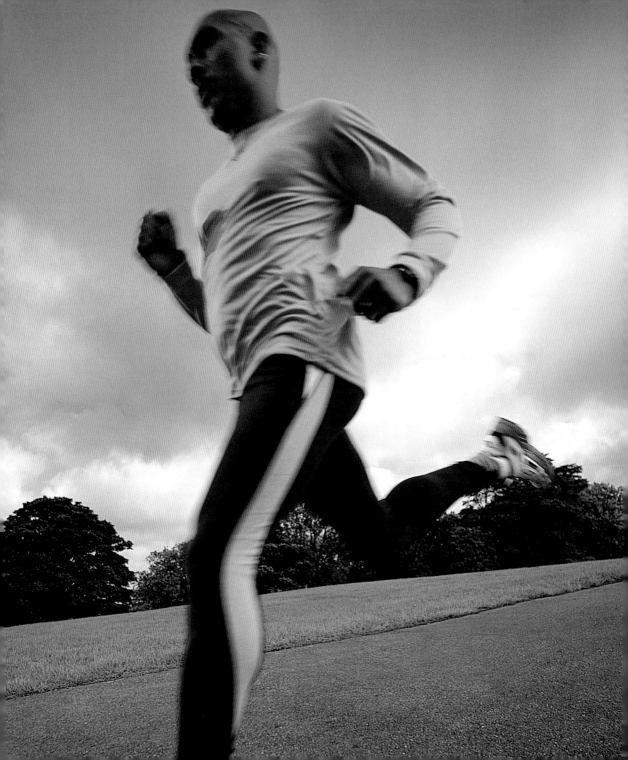

TABLE 1 Different body types and their characteristics
Mesomorphs
BODY CHARACTERISTICS ■ Usually tall with broad shoulders, narrow waists ■ 'V' shaped torso ■ Upright posture ■ Well muscled with good definition; fit and athletic ■ Can have fairly fast metabolism
FITNESS/SPORTS ADVANTAGES/SUITABILITY ■ Mesomorphs respond well to CV and resistance training, due to their adaptable and responsive physiology ■ They can sustain low body-fat levels ■ Both isolation (single) and compound (multi) muscle group exercises can be used to derive positive training adaptation (*see* page 64) ■ Depending on fitness/sports' needs, they will find it relatively easy to gain or lose weight ■ Can be freer with their food choices – but this does not mean eating unhealthily
FITNESS/SPORTS DISADVANTAGES ■ Mesomorphs can become over-trained and suffer from over-training (*see* page 101), as their bodies are quite robust when it comes to training. Their training therefore needs to be balanced, and mindful that consistent higher-intensity work must be moderated ■ They can put on weight quickly when they stop training ■ Their training needs to be progressive and constantly changing to prevent stagnation. This results from their ability to respond more quickly than the other two body types to training
Ectomorph
BODY CHARACTERISTICS ■ Small muscles, low body fat and wiry appearance ■ Medium to tall height ■ Fast metabolism – hence crucial need to *increase* calorie consumption to build and maintain muscle and training readiness; as such, they need to create a 'positive energy balance' – i.e. take in more calories than they burn (*see* page 106)

Ectomorph (cont.)

FITNESS/SPORTS ADVANTAGES/SUITABILITY
■ Light frame makes them suited to aerobic activity ■ Additionally, smaller body surface area also enhances their suitability for endurance activity, as their bodies are better at keeping cool

FITNESS/SPORTS DISADVANTAGES
■ Can achieve very low body-fat levels, which can be detrimental to health (below 6%)
■ Difficult to build muscle if participating in a sport that benefits from this, or for aesthetic reasons (but it can be achieved) ■ Can be more prone to injury, therefore need to follow a rigorous pre-conditioning programme (*see* page 38)

Endomorphs

BODY CHARACTERISTICS
■ Have large frames, with a 'strong' appearance ■ Unfortunately this can come with a high body fat percentage – most of it concentrated around the stomach giving them the (common for men) apple shape ■ Medium to tall ■ Can have fairly slow metabolism

FITNESS/SPORTS ADVANTAGES/SUITABILITY
■ Size benefits sports such as rugby and shot putting where bulk is useful as long as it can be moved powerfully ■ Often have large lung capacities which can make them suited to, for example, rowing (*see* page 45) ■ Can increase muscle mass much more easily than ectomorphs

FITNESS/SPORTS DISADVANTAGES
■ Their weight can make it difficult to perform sustained aerobic activity such as running, due to the impact forces involved and the stress this can place on joints ■ Can gain weight easily and lose condition quickly if training is ceased and calorie control not followed

The difference between body type and body shape

Body shape is the trained response or the everyday life response/effect that 'changes' an individual's body type. A long-distance runner may, for example, have a body type that has mesomorphic tendencies; however, while they are in training, due to their high calorie expenditure and lack of training emphasis on building (and maintaining muscle), they may well develop a more ectomorphic shape. Countless millions of people will take on more of an endo-morphic shape as they gain weight, due to a lack of exercise, too greater food consumption and poor dietary choices. To consider your body type, think back to your early adolescence and reflect on your shape then – if you trust your memory, you should 'see' a good indication of what your body type is.

How we shape up can depend on more than our body type

Although our body type will affect the way we respond to training, we should not become disillusioned or think that because we are not a particular type (more often than not meso-morphic) that we will not be able to achieve the fitness level or body shape we desire. There's a great deal more to how we shape up. The nature versus nurture approach provides one highly determining alternate factor, as does our genetic profile.

NATURE VERSUS NURTURE

Body types – as has been shown – are established at birth, but body shape is the result of physiological adaptations to training, diet and lifestyle. However, there are sufficient anomalies in sport, for example, to show that body types can vary between sports (within certain parameters) and playing positions. Compare, for example, the more endo-mesomorph body shape of Wayne Rooney with the more ecto-mesomorph Thierry Henry – both great football strikers. So, you should not throw your sporting or fitness aspirations out of the window because you don't think you have the perfect body type for your sport or fitness goals.

In many ways 'you are what you train for'. Nurture strongly shapes our fitness and sporting choices. So, within certain parameters, it will be possible to train for a specific fitness or sporting outcome regardless of body type, *and* achieve good results. OK, certain types may have an advantage over others when it comes to training adaptation and changes to body shape and sports performance, but this does not mean that because we are predisposed towards one type that we cannot 'move' it towards another. The crucial aspect is adhering to the right training plan and diet.

GENETIC PREDISPOSITION

Recently, research has begun to appear on fitness and sporting genes. Basically, genes have been discovered that are relevant to enhanced sports performance and fitness gains. In 2005 nearly 200 genes were identified as having an effect on sports and fitness performance and training adaptation.[i] The EPOR (erythropoietin receptor) gene, for example, has been identified as crucial for red blood cell production. In some people this gene mutates and continues to function, producing an abnormal amount of red blood cells. Finnish researchers identified an entire family with this EPOR mutation, several of whom were championship endurance athletes.[ii] As red blood cells are crucial for carrying oxygen to the working muscle, the EPOR gene is crucial for enhancing CV (aerobic) performance. Other similar genetic research has indicated that 1 in 5 Europeans cannot produce the alpha-actinin-3 protein found in speed- and power-producing fast twitch muscle fibres,[iii] making them less predisposed to power sports such as sprinting.

Thus, as with the nature versus nurture debate, we have another very strong influencing factor that can determine how our bodies shape up, although with the latter we will probably not know exactly how this will occur. I make these points to indicate that your body – regardless of type – may adapt differently to how you might expect, but you will not be aware of this until you start training.

Obesity and male health problems

In the UK, 66 per cent of men are either overweight or obese. This brings with it numerous potential health problems, such as osteoarthritis, heart disease, type 2 diabetes, high blood pressure, depression and cancers, such as that of the prostate. It has been calculated that this results in 30,000 deaths a year and a total cost to the country of £2 billion.

BEING OVERWEIGHT AND MALE: THE STATISTICS

- 6 out of 10 men in the UK are overweight
- 1 in 6 are obese
- The number of obese men has tripled in the last two decades.

---

[i] www.medscape.com/viewarticle/551096

[ii] www.newscientist.com/channel/life/genetics/mg19125655.300-only-drugs-can-stop-the-sports-cheats.html

[iii] www.newscientist.com/channel/life/genetics/mg19125655.300-only-drugs-can-stop-the-sports-cheats.html

As men, we are becoming as concerned about our appearances as women. At no other period in history has the pressure been so great to look good. Unfortunately, this has coincided with a time when we are fatter than ever. We see chiselled jaw lines and six-pack abs in our magazines, and while watching the latest action film, yet 6 out of 10 of us are over-weight and carrying too much fat. So what's the deal regarding fat?

Fat is a source of energy. It's one of the three

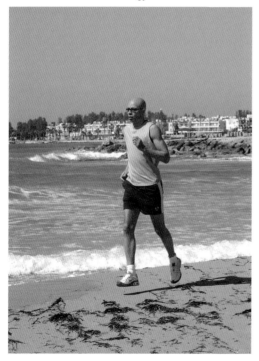

macro-nutrients – along with protein and carbo-hydrate (*see* Chapter 9). Fat is calorie dense when compared to the other macro-nutrients – containing about twice as many calories per gram (9 versus 4). What's not used for energy is stored in our bodies in various ways. Although we should not boast about it to our wives and girlfriends, we are much better genetically predisposed to having lower body-fat levels than them. But this also means that we have less of an excuse for having unhealthy levels (*see* healthy body fat guidelines page 113).

Men tend to carry the majority of excess weight around their stomachs, forming the stereotypical 'beer gut' apple shape. However, particularly overweight (obese) men will carry additional fat across their whole body. This will show too in the face, arms and legs.

To get an idea as to whether you are over-weight or underweight, you can use Body Mass Index (BMI) or waist measurement.

BODY MASS INDEX

Divide your weight in kilograms by your height in metres squared, and compare your result with the table on page 10.

Example: If you weigh 75kg and are 1.8m tall, your BMI would be 23:

$$\frac{75}{1.8 \times 1.8\ (3.24)} = 23$$

Table 2 BMI reference scores	
Type	**BMI**
Underweight	> 20
Ideal weight	20–25
Overweight	26–30
Obese	31–40
Grade 3 obesity	< 40

If your BMI is in excess of 31 you should contact your doctor.

There are limitations with BMI calculations. For example, if you are an athlete or fitness trainer and well-muscled, it is possible to have a BMI that indicates that you are overweight or obese when in fact you are not. This could particularly affect trained meso-endomorphs and endomorphs.

WAIST MEASUREMENT

Simply measuring your waist (around the belly button) can tell you much about your weight and your potential health issues. If your measurement is in excess of 94–102cm (37–40 inches), you are overweight, and if the measurement is in excess of the upper figure, then you are classified as being obese.

Carrying weight around your middle seriously increases your risk of heart disease and type 2 diabetes.

Body composition

Our bodies are made up of different types of tissue: lean body tissue and adipose (fat) tissue.

LEAN BODY TISSUE (FAT-FREE MASS)

Lean body tissue is made up of muscles, bones, blood and organs. This tissue is metabolically active, meaning that it requires and uses energy to function.

Muscle, for example, burns up to three times as many calories as any other part of the body. Every 0.45kg (1lb) gain will increase daily calorie burn by 30–50 calories. That may not sound a lot, but it can make a big difference as it does this each and every day. With that 0.45kg increase, you could burn an additional 350 calories a week, which is about the same amount as going for a moderate-intensity 30-minute run.

More information on fat as a nutritional source can be found on page 112.

> ### Training tip
>
> Weight training is not only crucial for improving our strength and mobility but is also key to improving our body shape and reducing body fat. This is because it makes our bodies much more effective everyday calorie burners.

FAT (OR ADIPOSE) TISSUE

This tissue is made up of the following components:

- Essential fat: this is stored in bone marrow, the heart, lungs and liver and other vital organs; it supports life.
- Storage fat: this acts rather like a cushion, protecting the body's vital organs. It is spread below the skin's surface (also known as subcutaneous fat).
- Non-essential fat: non-essential fat is just that; it's what makes us overweight or obese. It does not significantly fuel the body with energy (carbohydrate is the body's preferred activity fuel). It has no real purpose and is of course detrimental to our health if we store too much of it.

Body-fat testing

A body-fat (or body-composition) test can tell us whether our bodies have too much non-essential fat and what our lean (mainly muscle weight) is.

(The BMI test and waist measurement tests (*see* page 10) will provide an indication, but won't indicate lean versus fat weight.) There are various ways to measure body fat – for example, with bio-electrical impedance machines, callipers and calculations or underwater weighing. However, most of us will be able to tell if we are carrying too much non-essential fat simply by looking at our bodies.

If you do take a body-fat test (many gyms offer this service) and/or have a measuring kit at home, don't become overly concerned with the resultant body fat percentage reading or calculation – even if you are a serious sports performer. I believe it is far better to be concerned with training response and progress. Increased fitness will bring with it a host of positives, such as reduced risk of heart disease, lower stress levels, greater energy and improved body shape – as well as reduced body fat. Concentrating on body fat alone can be an unhealthy preoccupation (*see* eating disorders on page 13).

> ### Training tip
>
> In terms of training to change our body shape we should focus on the outcomes of our training: the fact that our CV fitness is improving or that we are getting stronger or faster, rather than focusing on how much body fat we have. It's a given that if our fitness improves, so too will our body composition and shape.

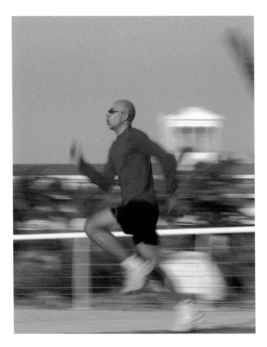

through lack of exercise or poor dietary control.

Up until quite recently it was thought that 'killing off' fat cells through working out and calorie controlled eating was impossible, but now exercise scientists believe we can get rid of fat cells permanently through a consistent exercise and dietary regime.

MALE BORDERLINE OBESITY EXPRESSED IN TERMS OF BODY-FAT PERCENTAGE		
Age	17–50	50+
Percentage	20%	25%

FAT CELLS

The body has billions of fat cells. These can become larger (fat cell hypertrophy) or can increase in number (fat cell hyperplasia)

HOW MANY FAT CELLS DO WE HAVE?	
Non-obese	25–30 billion
Moderately obese	60–100 billion
Massively obese	300 billion

Table 3 Acceptable body-fat levels for men	
Age	**Body fat**
21–30	12–18%
31–40	13–19%
41–50	14–20%
51–60	16–20%
61+	17–21%

If we attempt to reduce our body-fat levels any further than the lower figures indicated we run the risk of damaging our health. As you may have noted, I have indicated that men can relatively safely go lower than the figures indicated, to 6 per cent. However, this region is only for serious athletes – ectomorphic endurance runners, for example. Body-fat levels below 6 per cent will lead to health problems and a loss of libido.

Men and eating disorders

BEING UNDERWEIGHT

This is less common in men than being overweight. Ectomorphs will naturally be lean and wiry, with low body-fat levels. As I've indicated, the health risks for men in comparison to women are far less in terms of low body-fat levels. However, men (regardless of body type or shape) can suffer from eating disorders, such as anorexia or bulimia or traits of these.

An eating disorder is defined as 'having an obsessive interest in food and calories'. Anorexia is an eating disorder characterised by a fear of getting fat, not eating enough, excessive interest in food, and being fanatical about exercise. It can also involve the use of self-induced vomiting and laxatives. Bulimia shares similar traits to anorexia. However, it is characterised by swings between binge-eating and purging.

In sport and fitness activities an individual may become so preoccupied with his weight that he counts the number of calories in his meals and then calculates almost down to the last calorie how much exercise he needs to do to burn them off.

THE BIOLOGICAL AND PSYCHOLOGICAL REASONS FOR EATING DISORDERS

Biologically it is argued that neurotransmitters (chemicals that relay electrical signals between cells) in the brain are out of balance in those with eating disorders.

Psychologically there are numerous identified eating disorder traits, for example:

- Coming from a family that has difficulty expressing emotion and resolving conflict.
- Difficulties in coping with stress.
- Low self-esteem.

Anorexia and bulimia are psychiatric illnesses with specifically diagnosed traits. However, doctors have also defined 'sub-clinical eating disorders'. These are manifest in people who display some of the traits of the two eating disorders, and which may be detrimental to health and need addressing. These are likely to be found in sports and fitness participants (or those 'obsessed' with their appearance).

This is because these people are often subject to great external pressure to conform to a certain body shape and look; this can come from outside sources, but is very often from within. They may also become convinced that less weight and ridiculously low body-fat levels will bring them success.

EATING DISORDER WARNING SIGNS

- Preoccupation with food and calories.
- Feeling and expressing that you are fat when you are not.
- Indications (including smells) of vomit in the bathroom.
- Mood swings.
- Excess use of laxatives.
- Secret eating.
- Not wanting to eat in front of others.
- Having large weight swings in a short space of time.

Men who pursue extreme weight loss to improve sports performance, such as boxers, lightweight rowers or martial artists who have to make specific weight categories, can develop sub-clinical eating disorders. Their desire to 'make weight' by excessively restricting calories turns from being an end in itself to a means to an end.

Training tips

Avoiding sports- and fitness-related eating disorders

1 Have your dietary needs assessed by a nutrition expert. Research shows that those who control their own eating habits unsupervised are more likely to develop some kind of eating disorder.

2 Work with personal trainers and sports coaches who do not put unrealistic pressure on you to conform to a certain body shape or achieve unhealthy low body-fat levels.

3 Increase calorie consumption commensurately with increases in training volume.

4 If injured or ill, don't significantly reduce calorie consumption because you are not training. If you do this, you may not get all the nutrients you need to repair your injury or recover from your illness. Take expert advice.

5 Choose a fitness or sports activity that reflects your body type/current body shape. Doing this will prevent a possible 'mismatch' between your training and your aspirations for your body. To give an example, it would be unrealistic for an endomorph to achieve the slight frame of a distance runner.

If you think you (or someone you know) might have an eating disorder, then you should contact your GP. He or she will tell you where you can get help; many hospitals, for example, run specific clinics. You can also contact organisations such as the Eating Disorders Association (www.edauk.com).

Does body type influence your health?

Scientists have performed numerous studies to determine whether specific body types are more prone to certain diseases than others. One study involved 524 men (and 250 women) and the relationship between their somatotype and common diseases. Nearly 95 per cent of all the people in the survey fell into five somatotype categories. However, the most common somatotype for men was endomorphic/mesomorphic (large bodied, with heavy appearance). The researchers discovered that mesomorphic/endomorphs (larger, athletic bodies) frequently suffered from digestive system diseases, and that those with the highest levels of endomorphy and mesomorphy and the lowest ectomorphy suffered most from hypertension and liver disease – a likely consequence of them being overweight. This led the authors to conclude that having a 'dominant mesomorphy and marked endomorphy' was a risk factor in terms of predisposition towards certain diseases and requires

body weight control.[iv] This is a very important consideration when determining your body type and the type of training you should perform. Those with strong mesomorphic and endomorphic traits (who are not in regular training) could be best advised to initially perform workouts with a CV emphasis to burn calories, reduce body weight and improve heart health. Avoiding saturated fats and keeping fat consumption within acceptable levels is also crucial. (Note: These healthy tips apply to all body types.)

[iv] *Rev Environ Health*, 2002, Jan–Mar; 17(1): 65–84.

2 UNDERSTANDING YOUR BODY AND WORKING OUT

I've always been surprised by the number of guys who train but don't really understand what effects their workouts are having on their bodies. Failure to know how to target different muscle fibres and why higher-intensity workouts are better than lower-intensity ones, for example, can significantly impair the way you train your body type, how you attempt to change its shape, and how your body develops its fitness. In this chapter I provide an overview of the body's main physiological systems as they relate to men. Use this to contextualise the practical training information provided later.

The cardiovascular system, heart and lungs

The heart is a muscle, and it responds to aerobic (and anaerobic) training (see pages 18–19) in much the same way as a skeletal muscle such as the biceps does by growing in size and strength.

The key measures of the heart's efficiency are its stroke volume and heart rate. The former refers to the amount of blood the heart can pump around the body, and the latter refers to the effort that it has to put in to do so.

Heart rate is measured over a minute in beats per minute (BPM). It will decrease as a result of regular endurance training at sub-maximal exercise intensities. (Your maximum heart rate – HRMax – will remain largely genetically determined. HRMax refers to the maximum output of your heart.) Knowing your real or calculated HRMax (see page 50) will allow you to train safely and effectively in designated training zones, appropriate to your body shaping (or sports or fitness training goals, see page 57). Stroke rate is measured in litres of blood per minute.

A world-class endurance athlete or super-aerobically fit man's heart could pump 35 to 40 litres of blood around the body per minute and such a person may have a resting heart rate (RHR) of well under 50 BPM. (RHR describes the heart rate taken a few minutes after waking (see also page 10). It is a measure of increasing fitness.) This contrasts with an untrained individual whose heart may only be able to pump 20 litres or less, with a RHR of 75 plus.

MUSCLES AND CV TRAINING

It's important to realise that your heart, although the key determinant, is not solely responsible for improved CV fitness; this is because your oxygen transportation system, which includes your lungs, arteries, veins, capillaries and muscles, is an equally vital component.

Muscles, and in particular their constituent muscle fibres, will respond differently to the type of training they are subject to, with important consequences for body shaping and fitness and sports training. After a sustained period of CV training, the body will adapt and produce

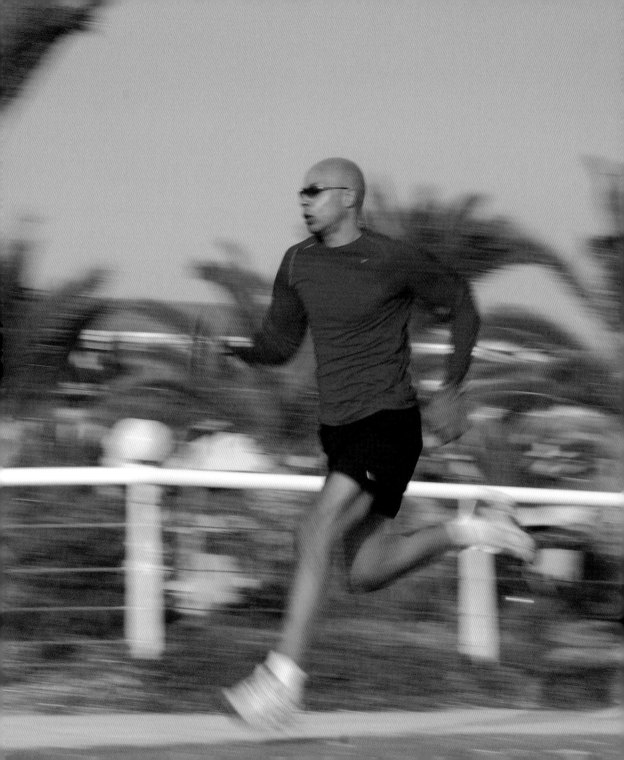

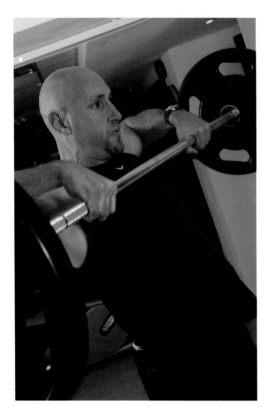

your muscle mass, but also emphasise aerobic (and tough anaerobic) training in your workouts, you will in all likelihood compromise your muscle building ambitions – of which more later.

The main exception are endomorphs who wish to shed fat and reveal their muscles – in their case, a high level of aerobic exercise is recommended (*see* page 47).

Energy systems

Our bodies are great machines and, like all machines, they need energy to power them. We can generate power through three 'energy systems'.

THE AEROBIC ENERGY SYSTEM

If you go for a steady, relatively easy-paced run you'll invariably be training aerobically. These workouts are often called 'steady state' because during them the body's energy demand is balanced by its energy supply, hence the steady state. In this situation our hearts are able to pump sufficient oxygenated blood around our bodies to fuel our aerobic engines.

Aerobic energy is produced when oxygen combines with glycogen (carbohydrate), proteins and fats and is broken down by enzymes in our muscles to generate energy.

more muscle capillaries. Capillaries can be viewed as oxygen-carrying highways – the greater their mileage, the greater the quantity of oxygen that can be transported to the muscles to fuel CV training.

Note that if you are an ectomorph (or have ectomorphic tendencies) and want to increase

Training tip

If your goal is increased muscle – whatever your body type – you should primarily use immediate anaerobic system training methods (*see* below) such as weight training with medium to heavy and heavy weights.

THE ANAEROBIC ENERGY SYSTEMS

If you've played football and had to chase back to make a tackle only to have to then sprint forward to provide an outlet for a mid-fielder to make a pass, you'll probably have first-hand experience of the anaerobic energy system. This type of high-intensity energy can only be sustained for relatively short durations. There are two anaerobic energy systems: the immediate anaerobic and the short-term anaerobic.

The immediate anaerobic energy system

The immediate anaerobic system has no reliance on oxygen and supplies explosive energy. This energy lasts no more than 10 seconds. It relies on stored energy sources – for example, creatine phosphate – in our muscles and a chemical reaction to fire it up. Lifting a set of weights or sprinting 40m are examples of this energy system in action. The first 10 seconds of any activity relies on the immediate anaerobic energy system.

THE SHORT-TERM ANAEROBIC SYSTEM

This energy system produces high-powered (but not flat-out) energy for up to 90 seconds. It also relies on stored energy sources, like the immediate system. A rally in tennis or a circuit training workout, or short burst of intense football or rugby, are examples of the short-term anaerobic energy system in action.

Under short-term anaerobic conditions, as the one and a half minute mark nears, oxygen takes on an increasing role in attempting to keep your body moving dynamically. After 30 seconds, 20 per cent of the energy produced is done so aerobically, and after 60 seconds it is 30 per cent. However, as the 90-second mark nears, no amount of oxygen gulping can breathe life into the short-term anaerobic engine, and it (and us) will grind to a potentially painful out-of-breath halt (this is due to a chemical reaction in our muscles and the formation of lactic acid.

Training tip

It is important to realise that aerobic and anaerobic training target different muscle fibres (*see* page 20), and because of this will strongly influence how our bodies 'shape' up.

Muscles and muscle fibre

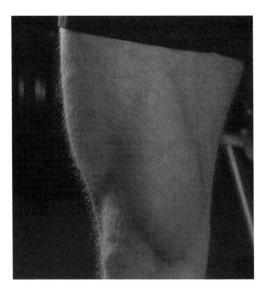

We have more than 430 muscles that we directly control, and over 250 million muscle fibres in the body. Muscle fibres are bundles of cells which are held together by collagen (connective tissue). In order to perform a sports skill or fitness activity, numerous muscles and muscle fibres interact. These are 'controlled' via electrical messages sent from the brain through the spinal cord and out to our muscles. When these signals reach the muscles, a chemical reaction results which causes the muscle to contract. Depending on the physical activity and the chemical reaction, this muscular action can be short-lived (anaerobic), or longer-lasting (aerobic), dependent on the energy system in use.

There are three main types of muscle fibre, and these respond differently to training. Knowing this fact is crucial to training your body type and altering your body shape.

SLOW TWITCH TYPE I FIBRE

Slow twitch Type I fibres are designed to sustain relatively slow, but long-lived muscular contractions. They are also known as slow twitch, red or slow oxidative (SO) fibres, as they can contract over and over again for long periods on aerobic energy. They twitch at a rate of 10–30 per second.

FAST TWITCH TYPE II FIBRE

Fast twitch muscle fibres contract two to three times faster than slow twitch muscle fibres, producing 30–70 twitches per second. These fibres are also known as white fibres.

There are two basic types of fast twitch fibre:

- Type IIa. Type IIa or 'intermediate' fast twitch fibres are also termed 'fast oxidative glycotic' (FOG) fibres because of their ability to display, when subject to the relevant training, a relatively high capacity to contract under conditions of aerobic and/or anaerobic energy production.
- Type IIb. Type IIb fibres are the 'turbochargers' in our muscles, they swing into

action for very high-power activities, such as a 40m sprint or heavy weight training workout. These fibres are also known as 'fast glycogenolytic' (FG) fibres. They rely almost exclusively on the immediate anaerobic energy system to fire them up. These are the fibres that any body type wanting to increase muscle size should concentrate on (*see* page 71 for methods of training these fibres, as they are the ones that will predominantly increase muscle size).

Training tip

To recruit (use) our fast twitch muscle fibres we need a strong mental input. These fibres are bundled together (in motor units) and are switched on (recruited) according to their size; the largest and most powerful ones need the greatest mental stimulation to get them working, unlike the smaller ones. This means that we need to be motivated and in the zone to fire them into action. This can result in an almost seamless stream of electrical impulses being sent to them from the brain, which produces optimum stimulation. Heavy weight training or sprint training will gather many of these large motor units together for action, but you must be in the zone to switch them on.

The endocrine system and its effects on body type

Training will have a significant hormonal effect on your body, which will significantly stimulate and affect adaptation. I didn't realise this until quite recently; just like many of you, I was focusing on the more mechanical outputs of my training, such as producing more powerful muscles, for my sport of choice: sprinting.

Hormones can be described as 'chemical messengers'. They are produced from a number of sites (endocrine glands) on the body (for example, the hypothalamus in the brain and the gonads); their major function is to change the rate of specific reactions in cells.

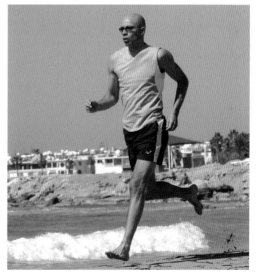

Our muscles (like the rest of our bodies) are composed of cells, and it is the way that certain hormones interact with these that is crucial to the way our body type will adapt and shape up in response to training. The two key hormones in this respect are growth hormone and testosterone. They are termed 'androgens' as they serve an anabolic (growth/stimulatory) function.

GROWTH HORMONE (GH) AND WORKING OUT

GH is released from the anterior pituitary gland in the brain soon after a workout starts. This hormone is often referred to as the 'fitness or sports hormone' because it is involved in numerous positive anabolic functions that will enhance the performance of our bodies. Specifically, GH contributes to bone, cartilage and muscle growth. This explains why it has been used as an illegal ergogenic aid in numerous sports.

TESTOSTERONE AND WORKING OUT

Testosterone is responsible for male sexual characteristics, but it also interacts with GH to augment its release. This makes it a powerful muscle builder. Testosterone also works with the

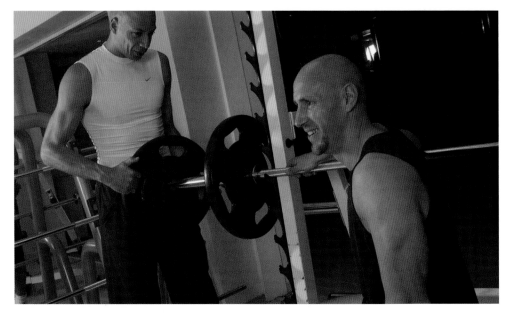

nervous system – an increased level could result in greater feelings of aggressiveness/dominance through 'interpretation' by the nervous system and brain. The mechanisms behind this process (and other hormonal influences on behaviour) are complex.

Both GH and testosterone release are affected by the intensity of our workouts and, more specifically, for example, even the weight training system used when weight training (*see* page 71).

Cortisol and working out

Cortisol is released from the adrenal gland; its levels are elevated by exercise. It stimulates protein breakdown, leading to energy production in the form of glucose from the liver. However, if it is your body-shaping aim to increase muscle size, this is not what you want, as amino acids (released via dietary protein breakdown) become preferentially used for energy rather than muscle building. This further explains why ectomorphs should avoid over-emphasising aerobic training if they are looking to build more muscle.

See page 116 for more information on protein.

Metabolic rate and body type

Metabolic rate refers to the energy that is released by the body to power all the processes needed to keep us alive and go about our daily lives. Working out can have a significant positive effect on metabolic rate and our body-shaping efforts (*see* page 88).

Metabolic rate is a matter of great debate when it comes to body types and weight loss. Many of us will blame our poor weight loss on a sluggish metabolism – and indeed, metabolic rate can be influenced by our body type. It is the case that those of us with endomorphic tendencies can have slower metabolisms. This results from greater fat storage on the body and potentially less lean muscle, which has a high metabolic cost. Fat is 'lazy' body tissue, and has little metabolic cost.

Metabolic rate is made up from:

- Total Daily Energy Expenditure (TDEE): This refers to the totality of all the energy the body burns over a day.
- Resting Metabolic Rate (RMR): A very significant proportion (60–75 per cent) of TDEE is used to maintain RMR. RMR encompasses

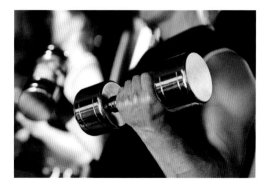

all those unseen and un-thought of essential bodily functions, such as heart, lung and mental functioning. Calculations of RMR are made over a 24-hour period, but do not include the calories burned while sleeping.

- Thermic Effect of Feeding (TEF): The process of eating and digesting food burns around 10 per cent of TDEE and is termed the TEF.
- Activity: Actual physical activity only accounts for about 15 per cent of TDEE, although this can be very significant in terms of affecting weight loss, weight gain, body composition and changing body shape.

How to calculate your metabolic rate

Step 1 Calculate your RMR

Age: 18–30   31–60

Multiply your weight in   Multiply your weight in
kg x 14.7 and add 496   kg x 8.7 and add 829

Example:

65kg individual   65kg individual
65 x 14.7 + 496   65 x 8.7 + 829
= 1451.5 RMR   = 1394.5 RMR

Step 2 Estimate your daily activity requirements in calories

Multiply your RMR by your daily activity level as indicated by the figures in the table opposite:

Activity level:	Defined as:	RMR Calculation
Not much	Little or no physical activity	RMR x 1.4
Moderate	Some physical activity, perhaps at work or the odd weekly gym visit	RMR x 1.7
Active	Regular physical activity at work and/or at the gym (three visits per week)	RMR x 2.0

Examples:

25-year-old weighs 65kg and has a moderate activity level – 1451.5 x 1.7 = 2466.7kcal
40-year-old weighs 80kg and has an active activity level – 1525 x 2.0 = 3050kcal

UNDERSTANDING ENERGY RELEASE FROM FOOD

Being guys, we often just pick up food products and toss them into the shopping basket as quickly as we can (if there is a shopping basket at the take-away!). Food labels may as well be written in hieroglyphics. However, it is important to consider the nutritional content of food products and understand their energy value.

kcal and calories

A kcal and a calorie supply the same amount of energy (that's why the terms can be used interchangeably).

Kilojoules

The kilojoule is the international standard for energy. 1kJ = 1000J. You'll see either or kJ and kcal on food labels.

A kJ is *not* the same as a kcal (or calorie) in terms of its energy provision. You can convert kJ into kcal and vice versa by using these calculations:

- To convert kJ into kcal divide by 4.2 – thus 200kJ = 48kcal (200/4.2)
- To convert kcal into kJ multiply by 4.2 – thus 100kcal = 420kJ (100 x 4.2).

Use the figures in Table 4 to gain an idea of how many calories you are burning during your workouts. Exercise (and other activity) calorie burning can have a significant effect on weight loss (or weight gain). *See* also post-exercise-induced calorie burning, page 88.

The figures in Table 4 are based on a 65kg man. If you weigh over this, you'll burn more calories; if you weigh less, you'll burn fewer calories. Also, as your fitness improves you'll also burn fewer calories at the same exercise intensity.

Men and ageing

Regardless of our body type, we will experience decline in our physical function with age.

Table 4 Energy costs of selected exercise methods

Activity	kcal/hour	Approx. kcal/min
Aerobics, high intensity	520	8.5
Boxing (sparring)	865	14.0
Cycling 16km/hour	384	6.4
Cycling 8.8km/hour	250	4.2
Rowing (moderate)	445	7.4

Table 4 Energy costs of selected exercise methods (cont.)

Activity	kcal/hour	Approx. kcal/min
Swimming (fast)	615	10.2
Weight training	270–450	4.5–7.5
Swimming for fitness	450	7.5
Treadmill running (5.6min/km)	750	12.5
Treadmill running (3.8min/km)	1000	16.6

Whatever our body type/body shape, those who remain active can seriously challenge this decline. I have provided some reasons for physiological decline and given you solutions below – the rest is up to you...

Training tip

There are 3500kcal in 0.45kg (approx. half a pound) of fat. Although this may sound an incredible number – when compared to the calories you could burn in a workout – regular training can make a big difference.

If you burned only 300kcal a day through your chosen exercise method, in a year you could theoretically remove 13.6kg of fat from your body.

1) SMALLER MUSCLES

We will all experience a 10 per cent decline in muscle mass between the ages of 25 and 50 and a further 45 per cent shrinkage as we reach our eighth decade if we do nothing about it. With decreased muscle comes reduced strength and power and reduced metabolic rate, and therefore a greater potential to gain weight. Also, we'll not look so good.

Solution: Weight (and resistance) train, maintain optimum protein and carbohydrate consumption and consider supplementing with creatine (*see* pages 128–9).

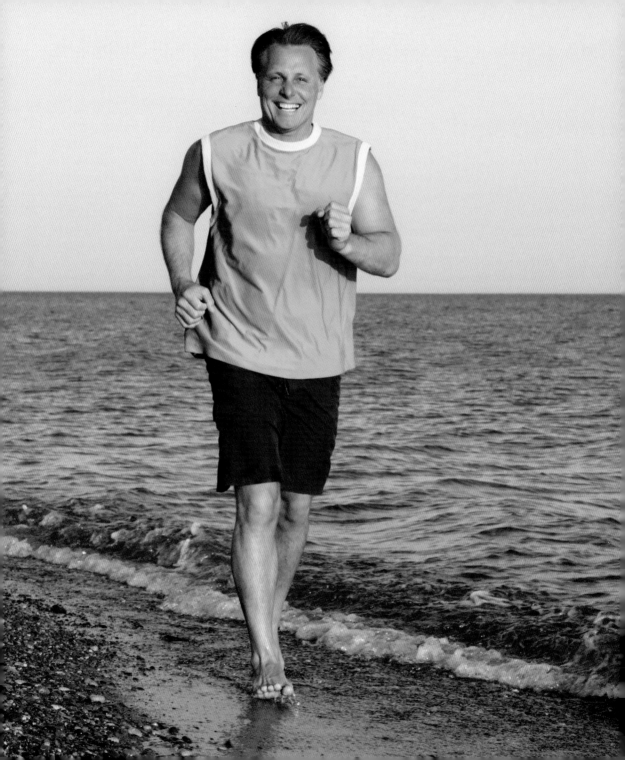

2) LESS GROWTH HORMONE

One of the major consequences of a reduction in growth hormone production is a diminished level of protein synthesis. As protein is the key building block for muscle, this also leads to muscle shrinkage with a consequent reduction in strength and power. Less GH will also make us feel less vibrant.

Solution: As for point 1, plus (where appropriate) intense and consistent training.

3) DECLINE IN FAST TWITCH MUSCLE FIBRE

Fast twitch muscle fibre declines much faster than slow twitch fibre with age – by as much as 30 per cent between the ages of 20 and 80. This is because the nerves that control these fibres die off, with knock-on consequences for the fibres themselves. This slows us down and reduces our strength.

Solution: As for points 1 and 2, plus some sports speed and power training (*see* page 71).

4) REDUCED PRODUCTION OF CREATINE PHOSPHATE

Creatine phosphate is one of the premium ingredients for short-term 'explosive' anaerobic physical activity (*see* page 19). Production of this body chemical declines with age, and with less of it in our muscles and less regenerative capacity, we'll have less energy for interval training and other stop-start activities such as football and tennis.

Solution: Performing stop-start (interval training) activities in training can return the creatine phosphate levels of older men to near those of young men.

5) REDUCED FLEXIBILITY

With age, soft tissue (muscles, ligaments and tendons) hardens and joints stiffen, increasing the potential for injury.

Solution: Regular stretching (*see* page 30).

Training tip

It does not matter how old you are, or what your body shape is, when beginning (or returning to) a workout programme as your body will always respond to training. Older men just need to be a bit more circumspect and use that 'wise head on your shoulders'.

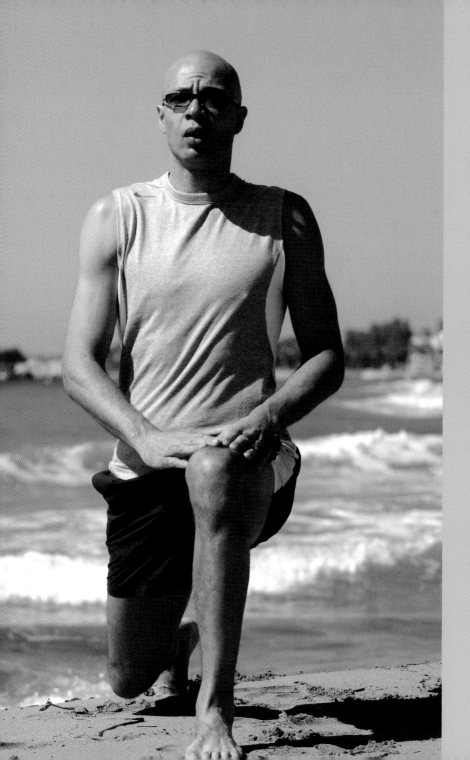

PART 2
TRAINING YOUR BODY TYPE

3 WARMING UP

After reading Part 1, you should be able to identify what body type you have, and what your current body shape is and some of the key physiological aspects that will affect your training. In this section of the book I show you how to get the most from your training for your body type and current shape. I have divided it into pre-conditioning (that's training to train, which will reduce potential injury), CV training, resistance training, and provided an overview of sports training and training planning. There's also information on the importance of using your mental muscle.

The majority of workout information provided is focused around two common male training goals: losing weight and gaining muscle. (In Part 3, I link these goals with relevant nutrition strategies and possible supplement use.) I start this part of the book, however, by looking at the important aspect of warming up.

Many guys don't like to stretch, favouring a much more direct approach to their workouts. Up until recently this approach would have been regarded as a bad thing, and potentially injurious. However, recent changes in thinking, backed up by sports science, have reduced the importance and relevance of stretching prior to most workouts. However, before you say 'I told you so', you still need to perform preparatory, more dynamic movements as part of your warm-up. And there is still a place for stretching.

Research indicates that stretching has no direct benefit to dynamic activities such as weight training or running – instead you need to 'dynamically' warm up.

Training tip

First the good news: you don't have to do lots of stretching before your workouts. Now the bad news: you still need to stretch. This should be done *after* your workouts to re-elongate muscles and aid recovery. And you should also stretch more regularly if you have any 'tight' areas that restrict perhaps the movement required for your sport or fitness activity, and/or are in middle or older age to counter the decline in flexibility that occurs as the years pass.

Stretching is more important if you are new to exercise

If you are just starting out on a workout programme, then stretching is important. It would obviously be inadvisable for an out-of-condition, overweight endomorph to begin his workout programme with a relatively high-intensity warm-up. Instead, time must be spent preparing his body for his workouts, and in this respect stretching is a must. Whether you are training for fitness or sport, your muscles must be able to attain safely the positions (range of movement) required for their safe and optimum performance. Strengthening the relevant muscles is equally important (*see* pre-conditioning, page 38).

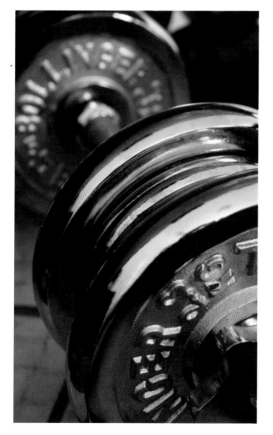

Yoga and Pilates

Although you may think that these activities are not for you, they can actually have very positive effects on your body shape and general training. Both activities require postural awareness and are great for core strength. Our posture is crucial for aesthetic and functional reasons – weak stomach muscles can lead to back problems, for example. Yoga and Pilates can do much to improve posture and strengthen weak areas. They can also re-energise and, as such, make a welcome break from your regular workouts. I've done both, and have used them accordingly as adjuncts to my athletic training. Once familiar with individual exercises, you can then incorporate some into your other workouts. Numerous other sportsmen incorporate yoga and Pilates exercises into their sports conditioning.

Hot (or Bikram) yoga is a great guy-oriented form of yoga, taking place in rooms heated to 40.5 degrees C and comprising 24 postures; this form of yoga develops strength and also has a significant CV effect. You'll also sweat a lot, and your heart rate will elevate as your body attempts to keep cool.

The 'new' way to warm up for fitness and sport

The key feature of the new more 'dynamic' warm-up is the incorporation of exercises that replicate the movement patterns and the speeds of movement of the exercise/exercises you are going to perform in the main part of your workout. As an example, if you are going to run, then your dynamic warm-up could contain walking lunges, high knee lifts, simulated running arm action movements, arm swings and calf raises. For weights workouts, although you may wish to incorporate some of these and other movements in your warm-up, the key is to perform warm-up sets of 8–10 repetitions at a light weight, prior to performing your designated reps, sets and weight to be lifted on the exercise you are going to perform in the main part of your workout.

Dynamic warm-ups will optimally prepare your body for the similar activity to follow. Static stretches, such as bending forward and down to touch your toes, have little direct relevance to fitness and sports activities as part of the warm-up. They involve a different type of muscle contraction (*see* page 20) to the one that your muscles will be put through when you actually work out. Note, as previously mentioned, there are some exceptions when you should stretch, such as if you are suffering from tightness in a body part/parts as a result of a focused period of training. To provide an actual example: the forearms and lower back may become tight after repeated rowing workouts and require some static stretches to loosen them before rowing and between workouts. On a more everyday basis, you may have had a hard day in the office and be suffering from a stiff back and a good stretch can relax and energise (see top of the world stretch page 44, for a good remedial static stretch).

Suitable dynamic warm-up exercises for selected fitness activities

ROWING

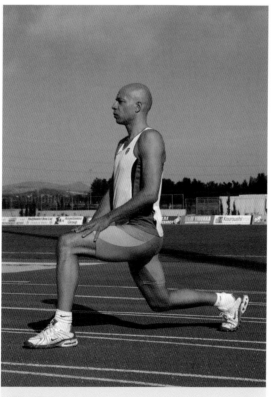

Fig. 3.1 *Lunges*

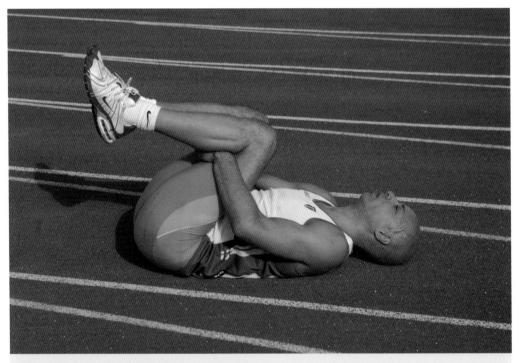

Fig. 3.2 *Lower back stretch*

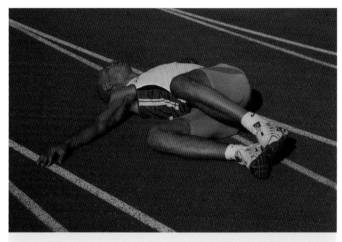

Fig. 3.3 *Lying side-to-side trunk rotations – right*

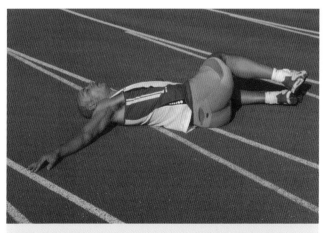

Fig. 3.4 *Lying side-to-side trunk rotations – left*

RUNNING
(Also use lunges and side-to-side trunk rotations from pp. 33 and 35.)

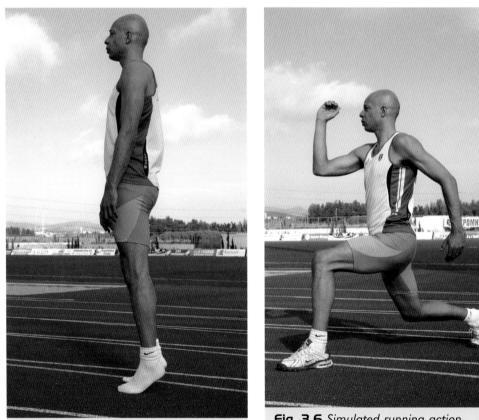

Fig. 3.5 *Calf raises*

Fig. 3.6 *Simulated running action with arms*

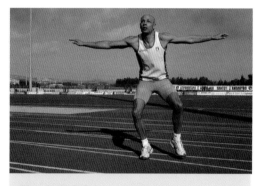

Fig. 3.7 *Sideways running*

For sports: The dynamic warm-up should include exercises similar to those identified in pp. 33–6, plus those specific to the particular sport – for example, simulated kicks without a ball for football and rugby players.

For these and other similar activities, 5 minutes of gentle CV exercise should be performed first. This will turn on the myriad of physiological processes needed for an effective workout. With weight training there is less need for CV preparation. However, after CV and resistance workouts, you should cool down with some gentle CV activity and perform some stretches on the muscles you have targeted. Hold these for 15 seconds.

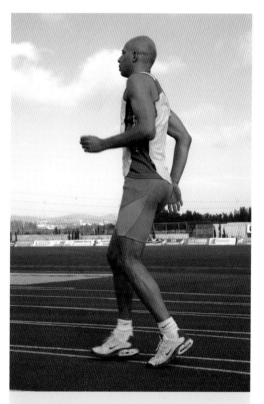

Fig. 3.8 *Backwards running*

4 TRAINING TO AVOID INJURY (PRE-CONDITIONING)

Although pre-conditioning (or pre-training) derives from the world of sports training, its philosophy and practice are just as important for 'everyday' fitness training, whatever your body type/shape. Basically, pre-conditioning is the training you do to significantly reduce injury and deal with any previous injuries. It runs consistently in the background to your main workout programme.

Why pre-condition?

Ectomorphs or those with ectomorphic tendencies can be prone to strain injuries due to their lighter frames. However, they could reduce the chances of joint injury, for example, by following a suitable pre-conditioning routine. Relevant exercises would include leg extensions and leg curls and eccentric calf raises to bolster their soft tissue against injury.

As an example close to home, I suffer from sore Achilles tendons brought on through years of sprint training (this is also a common complaint among runners of longer distances). This affects both tendons from time to time – on numerous occasions it has prevented me from training. However, I always try to keep the potential problem in check by performing relevant pre-conditioning exercises, such as heavy weight eccentric movement calf raises and balances. These exercises strengthen the calf muscles and Achilles tendons and reduce potential strain.

To perform the former exercise (and other similar eccentric muscle strengtheners) the emphasis is placed on the lowering phase of the movement using a slow five-count. This downward movement improves the shock absorbency of muscles and tendons.

An eccentric muscular contraction occurs when a muscle 'lengthens as it contracts'. They are absorbent and controlling contractions. As an example, they occur in the calf, thigh and hip muscles when running on the flat, but particularly downhill. Most physical activity emphasises concentric contractions. These occur when a muscle shortens as it contracts, as during the lifting phase of a biceps curls in the biceps muscle.

Regardless of body type or shape, your training programmes should train muscles concentrically and eccentrically (*see* also page 67).

What should you incorporate into your pre-conditioning programme?

It is impossible to provide an answer for everyone, but I'd recommend that you speak to a personal trainer, relevant sports coach or physio. Explain to them what training you are doing, what your training history and injury history is, and they should then be able to select appropriate exercises for you. They should, of course, reference your body type and current shape.

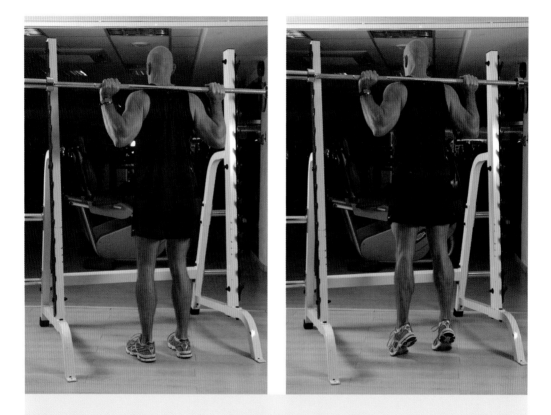

Figs. 4.1 a and b *Performing pre-conditioning exercises, such as the eccentric calf raise, will reduce the potential for disrupted training – regardless of body type.*

Selected pre-conditioning exercises related to fitness and sports activities

LEG EXTENSION (WEIGHTS)

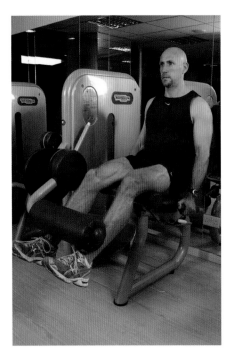

Gradually increase the weight lifted to a medium to heavy weight, performing 2–4 sets of 6–10 repetitions with one minute's recovery between sets.

Pre-conditioning value

Stabilises and strengthens the knee joint – great if you're overweight or endomorphic and involved in running-based activities.

Fitness and sports applicability

All.

Comments/tips related to body type/ shape

- Suitable for independent left and right leg training for more balanced strength development.
- Of use to all body types/shapes to reduce impact related stresses on the knee.

(Note: Overweight men are best advised not to emphasise impact-based CV methods, such as running, in their training programmes to reduce potential joint stress.)

BACKWARD AND SIDEWAYS RUNNING (BODY WEIGHT)

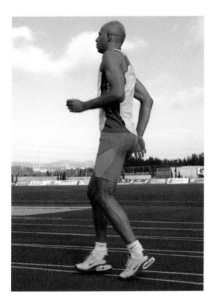

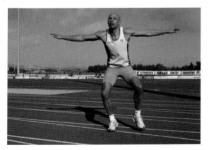

Perform over 10–20m, 4 times, building up speed as confidence and fitness improves.

Pre-conditioning value
Improves agility, lower limb strength, flexibility and balance and body awareness.

Fitness and sports applicability
Great for running/jumping-based sports, plus numerous others, such as skiing and snow boarding.

Comments/tips related to body type/shape
Can be included as a regular warm-up element – see dynamic warm-up (*see* page 31).

ECCENTRIC CALF RAISE

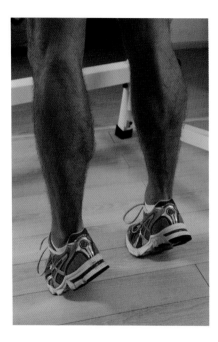

Perform 2–4 sets of 6–12 repetitions.

Pre-conditioning value
Strengthens Achilles tendons.

Fitness and sports applicability
Running and all running-based sports.

Comments/tips related to body type/ shape
All body types could benefit from this exercise as Achilles problems are common among sports and fitness trainers.

Training tip

Many guys think that more is better and can get well and truly bitten by the exercise bug. To make sure it does not bite you back, you must schedule rest periods into your training. If you don't, you run the risk of injury and illness and compromised training gains.

It is during recovery when the body adapts and grows stronger – not during training, this is why recovery and optimum nutrition is crucial (see Part 3).

An introduction to training planning is provided in Chapter 8.

THE PLANK

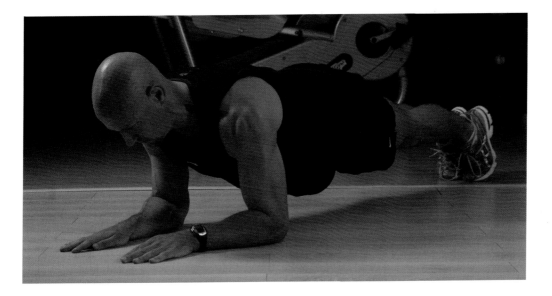

Increase the length of the hold from 5 seconds to 60 and beyond as confidence and fitness improves. Do 2–6 reps.

Pre-conditioning value
Strengthens the core.

Fitness and sports applicability
All fitness and sports activities.

Comments/tips related to body type/ shape
Back problems are common in both the fitness and sports worlds. The plank will develop core 'holding' strength, reducing the potential for injury when running or performing overhead weight lifting movements and those involved in everyday life. The exercise is suitable for all body shapes.

TOP OF THE WORLD FIT BALL STRETCH

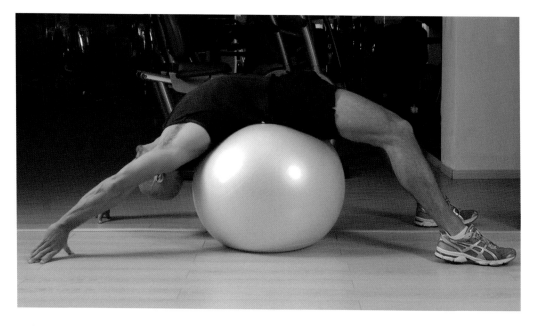

Hold the stretch for 20 seconds and do 3 reps.

Pre-conditioning value

Stretches the whole body from tip to toe. Counteracts the pulling forward emphasis of desk work and driving, and an over-emphasis on developing the muscles to the front of the body often caused through inappropriate exercise selection when weight training.

Fitness and sports applicability

All fitness and sports activities.

Comments/tips related to body type/shape

This exercise is suitable for all body shapes.

5 CARDIOVASCULAR TRAINING

As mentioned previously, I have geared the practical content of this book towards two key training goals for men of all body types and body shapes: gaining muscle and losing weight. Many guys will use CV kit for the latter reason, having identified it quite rightly as a great calorie burner. Note that although muscle tone will improve with CV training, it will not shape and build your muscles in the way that weights (and other resistance training methods) can (*see* page 65).

Health benefits of CV exercise

The key one is improved heart health.

A more muscular heart will be able to pump more oxygenated blood around the body with less effort. And this will, of course, reduce your risk of heart disease and lessen stress.

CV training and body types

ECTOMORPHS

As an ectomorph or ecto-mesomorph, your light body makes you suited to CV activities and in particular running – although you must always pre-condition (*see* page 38) to reduce injury potential. If you want to capitalise on your body type, then this is the way to go as training gains and adaptation will come relatively quickly. However, if you also want to increase your muscle size, then you have a more serious challenge on your hands. Your body will be walking a metabolic tightrope as CV training burns calories and potentially reduces your already low amount of muscle mass and increases your already high metabolic potential (*see* page 23). This will compromise your weight training attempts to build muscle (strategies to overcome this are presented in more detail on page 57).

MESOMORPHS

Mesomorphs adapt easily to most types of training; however, if they are more endomorphic (or overweight), then certain CV activities involving impact forces need to be carefully monitored and introduced into a training programme. This is because their heavier weight could lead to greater potential for joint injuries, notably to the ankles, knees and back. I would recommend indoor rowing as a great CV choice for mesomorphs (and endo-mesomorphs) and the overweight. Rowing engages more muscle than running, involving the legs, back and arms, and it is also load bearing. A look at top-class rowers, such as James Cracknell and Matthew Pinsent, readily indicates how the activity suits large (in fact, *very* large) guys. Bigger men often have naturally large lung capacities, which makes them genetically predisposed towards a CV activity such as rowing.

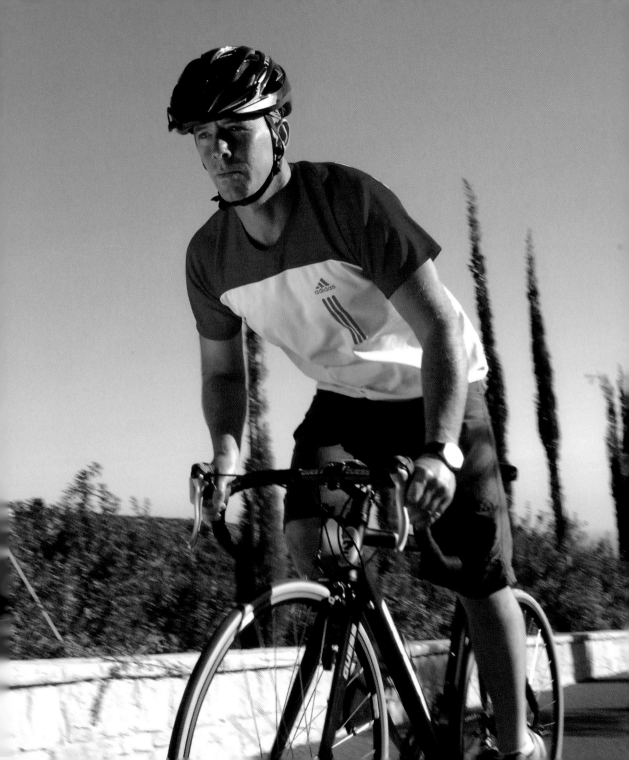

ENDOMORPHS

As I have indicated, having an endomorphic (or meso-endomorphic) body type can make certain CV activities less suitable, as can being overweight. These body types, with their naturally higher levels of muscle mass and larger frame, are more suited to strength and power-oriented fitness and sports activities, such as weight training, weight lifting and rugby. If you are an endomorph and want to CV train, perhaps for heart health or weight loss, then, as I previously mentioned, rowing would make a highly suitable activity. Cycling could offer similar benefits. This is not to say that running is to be avoided; rather, its use must be moderated by meso-endomorphs, endomorphs and the overweight due to the resultant impact strain that can be placed on the body. Walking before you progress to running is a great way to begin burning calories (*see* page 10).

Training tip

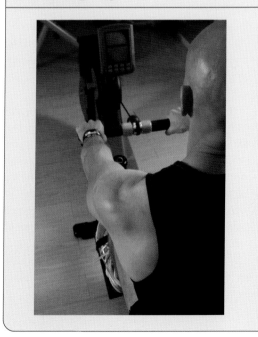

We guys often like to be competitive, so why not try the sport of indoor rowing? Training for an event or a time-trial to see how we rate against our peers, or just ourselves, can provide focus and great motivation for training. Most competitions take place over 2000m. The rowing machine manufacturer Concept2 is largely behind their organisation in the UK and worldwide.

There is a thriving online community with sites such as www.concept2.co.uk providing race details, forums and loads of training advice. Note if you become an 'ergonaut' you'll have to like pain, as rowing the 2km distance taxes the body like no other activity. I should know – it took me 45 minutes to stand up after one race! Rowing machines can be called ergometers – hence the term.

VO$_2$Max and body type

VO$_2$Max is a measure of lung capacity – put simply, it measures the amount of oxygen your lungs can process at maximum output. VO$_2$Max is measured in ml/kg of body weight per minute.

In the world of sport, multi Tour de France winning cyclist Lance Armstrong had a VO$_2$Max of 80–85ml/kg of body weight per minute. The untrained individual's VO$_2$Max could be less than half this. Specialist equipment is required to test VO$_2$Max and very few gyms offer this facility. However, an increasing number of heart rate monitors have a fitness facility that predicts your maximal oxygen uptake.

Interestingly – and with relevance to body types – VO$_2$Max is largely genetically inherited and can only be improved slightly through training. Mesomorphs and endomorphs can have very high natural VO$_2$Max capacity – they have large rib cages, which offer space for large oxygen-processing lungs. As we noted previously, rowing – because it is zero impact – can offer larger body types the chance to excel at an endurance activity. You don't have to be an ectomorph to have a great endurance body.

How to monitor your heart rate

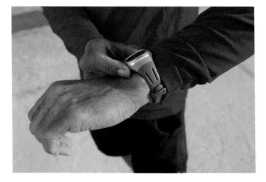

Whatever your body type, knowing how hard your heart is working can significantly influence how your body shapes up and how motivated you are to maintain a workout programme. Knowing this will also enable you to train within specific training zones that have specific effects on your body's adaptation – see Table 5.

Your heart rate will increase (in beats per minute) the harder you exercise. However, the fitter you are, the more efficient (and stronger) your heart will be (*see* page 16, stroke volume and heart rate). This will mean that you'll be putting in less effort to complete your CV workouts, everything being equal. It also explains why it is important to know what training zone you are in and what effect it is having on your body. This will leave you safe in the knowledge that you are developing a certain type of CV fitness practically and systematically. To this end I recommend that you purchase a heart rate monitor (although you can use specific calculations that allow you to estimate your workout effort – *see* box).

Training tip

Heart rate monitoring equipment
You might decide you want the most '*specced*-up' model, with features such as GPS and an altimeter, but in reality you probably won't use these or half the other features on offer. A base model will more than likely serve your needs (and these now offer a great deal). Really all you need your heart rate monitor to do is measure your heart rate, be able to establish training zones, and store this data for later analysis and download.

Table 5 Heart rate training zones

Heart rate %HRMax	Heart rate training zone and description
50–60	'Light to moderate' – for the older and untrained. Low-calorie-burning potential. Primarily works slow twitch muscle fibre. Energy created exclusively aerobically.
60–70	'Everyday fitness zone' – this zone enables relatively comfortable and sustained CV exercise to be completed. It is often associated with the misleading belief that it is the best for fat burning – the reasons why this is *not* the case are explained on page 52. This zone also largely targets slow twitch muscle fibre. Also used as a recovery zone for those with advanced levels of CV fitness. It has a moderate- to high-calorie-burning potential. Energy is created virtually exclusively aerobically.

Table 5 Heart rate training zones (cont.)	
Heart rate %HRMax	**Heart rate training zone and description**
70–85	'Quality aerobic training zone' – this is the zone for intermediate and advanced trainers. It offers optimum calorie-burning potential for fat loss and great CV fitness development. Although the zone predominantly targets slow twitch muscle fibre, towards its upper end, with increased energy expenditure, it also involves fast twitch fibre, particularly Type IIa. These fibres will adapt and contribute towards generating increased CV power. This zone marks the transition into anaerobic training territory and can have a potentially significant post-exercise calorie-burning effect (*see* page 88).
85–100	'High intensity training zone' – this zone is for advanced trainers and competitive athletes. It's not possible to exercise in it for long. All muscle fibre types are involved. It can burn proportionally high numbers of calories for its short duration, although this is largely attributable to its effect on elevating post-exercise calorie burning. The upper end of this training zone really emphasises anaerobic energy production and targets fast twitch muscle fibres.

Calculative methods for establishing heart rate maximum and training zones

You'll probably be aware of the '220–your age' method of calculating your maximum heart rate (HRMax). You might also know that this formula can be inaccurate, by 10–15 per cent. This is because HRMax can be affected by stress, heat, hydration, fitness, motivation and even type of CV exercise – readings will invariably be higher on a rowing machine or treadmill and lower on a step machine or cycle due to the greater amount of muscle involved in generating energy on the former kit. Recently, a new calculative formula has been recommended as being much more accurate than the '220–your age' one.

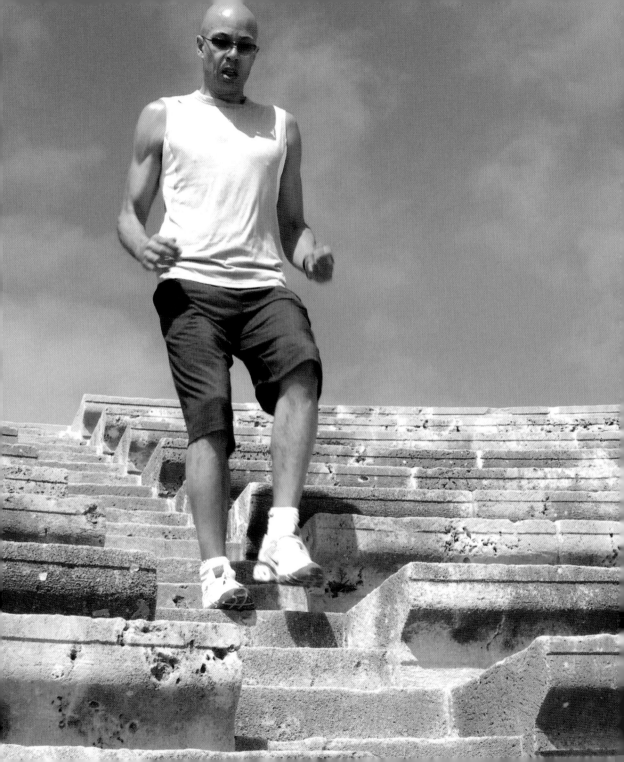

For simplicity, this uses the following calculation: 207 – 0.7 x your age).[v] Using this formula, the predicted HRMax for a 30-year-old would be 186 (this would compare with 190 using the 220 – your age formula).

WHY DO YOU NEED TO KNOW YOUR HRMax?

As indicated, knowing your HRMax, calculated or actual, enables you to train within designated heart rate zones.

Only advanced CV trainers should perform a HRMax test – this requires incremental increases in exercise intensity, usually over 2-minute periods, until exhaustion is reached. At this point HRMax is achieved and measured.

Burning fat – there's no real fat burning zone

The fat burning zone (FBZ) is used to refer – although (encouragingly) less frequently these days – to relatively low-intensity CV workouts that last for more than 20 minutes. Unfortunately, the concept of the FBZ is misleading and could result in you exercising ineffectively for optimum weight loss for your body type.

The idea of a specific FBZ developed because 1) CV workouts carried out at a moderate inten-sity are both sustainable and achievable by those new to exercise, and 2) lower-intensity CV workouts seemingly burn more fat calories. You'll see from Table 6 that at a low exercise intensity, 66.6 per cent of calories are derived from fat and 33.4 per cent from carbohydrate. Armed with this information, it's not too hard to see how low-intensity CV exercise as advocated by the FBZ can be championed as the best fat burner. However, in reality fat burning and attaining a negative/balanced energy balance is best accomplished by training at higher CV intensities. This is because total calorie burn is what really counts (plus at these intensities a significant number of calories will be burned post-workout, as your body returns to steady state).

Calculating your energy expenditure

As many of us will be training to reduce body fat, working out the energy spent during a workout will be important. Although men are perhaps less into calorie counting than women, knowing how much energy 'we have left in the gym' is important when it comes to creating the 'negative energy' balance required to lose weight. Most heart rate monitors and CV kits offer calorie-counting functions – although useful, these provide estimates. I have also provided calorific expenditure for selected exer-

[v] *Med Sci Sports Exerc*, 2007, May; 39(5): 822–9.

Table 6 Percentage calories burned between fat and carbohydrate

Exercise intensity	Percentage of kcal from		Energy expenditure (kcal)	
	Carbohydrate	Fat	Per min	After 20 mins
Low	33.4	66.6	9.6	192
Medium	50.7	49.3	12.2	244
High	84	16	15	300
Very high	100	0	20.2	404

cise modes on page 25. *See* also page 24 for how to calculate your daily energy requirements, pages 144–149 for sample energy costs of selected foods, and page 88 for post-exercise calorie burning – all these factors are crucial when it comes to losing (or gaining) lean weight. Using this information you will be able to work out how many calories you need to create a negative (weight loss), positive (weight gain) energy balance or maintain your weight (balanced energy balance).

Training tip

Whatever your body type, that flat belly or elusive six-pack will probably still remain elusive if you don't do some CV work and cycle your training (see training planning). You'll need the CV work to burn additional calories and reduce body fat and a systematic but varied training programme to maximise training adaptation and prevent stagnation.

Training tip

Interval training

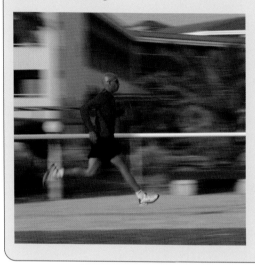

Interval training divides periods of effort between periods of rest. You could, for example, complete 3 x 5-minute intervals on a rowing machine with 2 minutes' gentle rowing recovery between each interval. The speed at which you complete the intervals will be determined by your fitness level and training goals. Interval training is suitable for all body types and shapes. You'll see from the selected workouts in Table 7 that I have designed some interval workouts for those new to exercise. These low-intensity workouts enable large chunks of exercise to be completed in one session, which would not initially be possible in one hit – given starting levels of fitness.

Burning up more calories with your feet

You'll probably like the sound of this. It works if you CV train regularly three to four times a week as your metabolic rate can be elevated by as much as 20 per cent – which means more calories being incinerated. This is the result of what's known as excess post-exercise oxygen consumption (EPOC). Basically, when we perform a CV workout our body switches on and turns up numerous physiological processes, notably oxygen processing and consumption to power our exercise efforts. Other related functions include the release of energy from muscle cells and the release of specific hormones, such as GH and testosterone. These processes do not return to base line levels immediately after a workout; instead, they continue operating at a high level as they return to a steadier state. Research identifies two EPOC phases: a very high-intensity one in terms of energy cost in the two hours immediately after a workout, and another of lesser intensity that lasts a further 48 hours. With regular training, this adds up to increased calorie burning all day and every day.

All body types will 'turn up' their metabolic rate with regular CV (and resistance) training (*see* page 62), which will benefit any desired weight loss goals. You should factor this in when calculating your 'energy balance' needs for weight loss or weight gain goals, specifically your activity expenditure.

Ectomorphs/ecto-mesomorphs, with their higher natural metabolic rates, will need to be particularly mindful of EPOC when performing regular CV work if they want to increase muscle mass. This is because their high metabolic rate will be significantly boosted by post-workout calorie burning. In

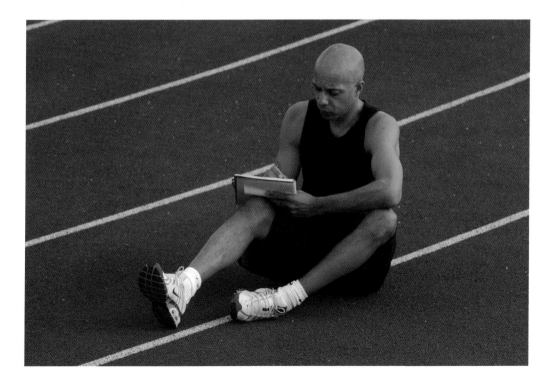

respect of this they will need to seriously consider their food consumption levels in order to create the positive energy balance needed to build more lean muscle (*see* page 106). This could mean, for advanced 5–6 days-a-week training ectomorphs, adding another 500 plus calories a day to their food consumption. Using supplements (*see* page 128) may be beneficial in this respect.

POST-EXERCISE CALORIE BURNING – A PERSONAL EXPERIMENT

If you don't believe me about calorie burning with your feet up, take a look at this. I set about testing the EPOC theory by doing a largely anaerobic interval-based track workout. It only lasted about an hour, including warm-up and cool-down, and involved just a couple of minutes of fast running with short recoveries. I kept my heart rate monitor on and referenced its calorie counting function. In the three hours after the workout it estimated a further 700 calories burned, compared to the 400 during the actual workout. Therefore 1100 calories were burned in total from an hour's workout. This is a significant amount; for inactive men, this is close to half of their daily calorie requirements. To stop me losing weight I would have to consume a similar number of calories.

EPOC is also created by weight training (*see* page 62).

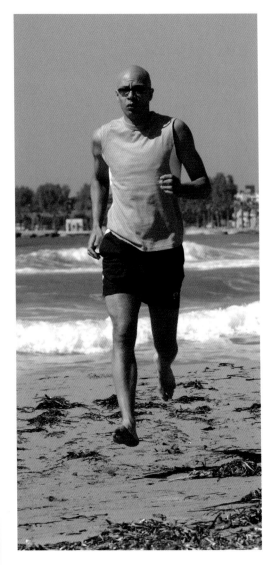

Table 7 Sample CV training plans for selected body types and training goals

Body type	Training experience	Training goals	Suggested workouts	Comment
Ectomorph	Intermediate	To build muscle and promote general health	**1)** Cycling 20 mins EDFZ **2)** Running 10 mins QAZ	You'll be primarily concerned with increasing muscle mass through your weights workouts, so the CV sessions are designed to contribute to heart health. If doing weights and CV in the same workout, always do your weights first, so you can give them more energy. (Note: To gain muscle, ectomorphs or ecto-mesomorphs will need to keep aerobic work to a minimum).
Mesomorph	Intermediate	Achieve high-end CV fitness and enter a 2km indoor rowing competition	**1)** 30 mins rowing, QAZ (mid- range around 80% HRMax) **2)** 60 mins rowing, EDFZ **3)** 3 x 8 mins rowing, higher range QAZ (85–90% HRMax average), with 3 mins easy rowing recovery between	This body type can train relatively hard without too many problems, when a reasonable level of fitness has been attained. To move up to the 'advanced' level the recoveries used should be reduced (where appropriate) and rowing speed increased, while remaining within the heart rates required of the training zones.

Table 7 Sample CV training plans for selected body types and training goals (cont.)				
Body type	**Training experience**	**Training goals**	**Suggested workouts**	**Comment**
			4) 6 x 1 mins rowing HIZ (95% HRMax) with 2 mins easy rowing recovery	
Overweight endo-morph/ meso-endo-morph	New to exercise/ returning after long lay-off	Weight loss and improved muscle tone	**1)** 45 mins walking EDFZ **2)** 2 x 7 mins cycling mid QAZ (75–80% HRMax) with 4 mins walk rest between intervals **3)** 20 mins cycling EDFZ	As this body type will be new to exercise, they will need to progress gradually and avoid stressing their joints. Workout 2 is a more intense one, but the interval format should allow for it to be completed. This is an early way to introduce a higher-intensity workout into a new-to-exercise routine. As fitness improves, the rest period can become increasingly active, with low-intensity CV work performed between intervals.

Guide to training zones (*see* **page 49 for details**)
EDFZ = everyday fitness zone
QAZ = quality aerobic training zone
HIZ = high-intensity zone

Training tip

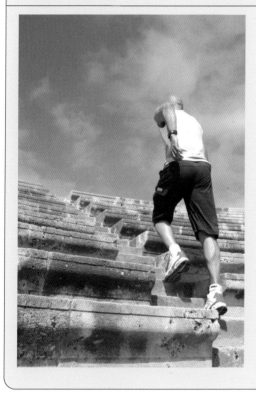

The higher your exercise intensity, the greater the potential for training and body shaping adaptation, everything else being equal – this is a consequence of the 'hit' on your metabolism and elevated androgen hormone release (*see* page 22).

(Note: Regardless of body type (although mesomorphs will have a potentially greater resilience), the use of very high-intensity sessions should be moderated in your training plans. Those new to exercise should obviously build up their fitness over a matter of months before tackling them. Don't think that training hard all the time is the best strategy; your body will eventually resent this and fail to adapt as effectively as it would if you scheduled in easy- and medium-intensity workouts, rest days and longer rest periods. You also run the risk of injury if you adopt such an 'eyeballs out approach'. (The importance of rest is covered in more detail on page 84.)

Training tip

If you are overweight, older or an endo-morph, don't be afraid to walk your way to CV fitness. Take a look at these calorie-burning statistics:

Walking speed	Gradient Calorie burn/hour			
	Flat	4%	8%	12%
4.2km/hour	270	391	526	662
6.4km/hour	400	579	759	930
8.0km/hour	530	769	979	1200

Average normal walking pace is 3.2 to 4.8km/hour.

Figures are based on an 80kg man. You will burn more calories if you weigh over this, and fewer if you weigh less.

The importance of 'correct' nutrition for CV training

■ Antioxidants (vitamins A, C, E and the minerals selenium and zinc, for example). These can reduce the cellular damage created by CV work (*see* page 122 for more information on antioxidants), although recent research indicates that this may be less important among experienced CV exercisers.

■ Hydration. Water (for workouts lasting up to an hour) or sports (energy) drinks (for workouts longer than an hour) will optimise your CV training.

■ Carbohydrate. This is needed to keep your muscle fuel (glycogen) stores stocked. Start this process immediately after your workout.

■ Protein. This is needed to maintain muscle mass. If you only do cardio, then you should go for 1.6–1.8g a day per kg of body weight.

Detailed nutritional advice and strategies as they relate to body type are provided in part 3.

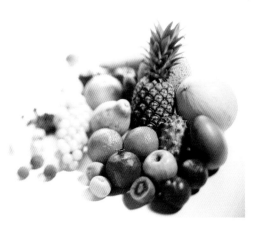

Training tip

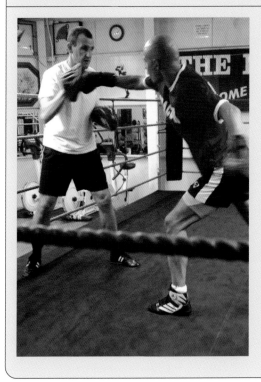

Find an exercise class for your body type, current body shape and fitness level

We guys may be a little unsure about venturing into the aerobics studio. This area may seem a bit too 'women only'. However, I'd advise you to take a look at the studio timetable, as you'll probably find a class that suits your level of fitness and your body type and shape – and is also fun. The options are virtually endless with new concepts and hybrid classes appearing all the time. Group CV classes, for rowing and running, are excellent ways for guys to train in a group to controlled heart rates. Boxing and martial arts-based classes are equally worth a go – they provide a great (if sometimes tough) way to build aerobic and anaerobic fitness, while yoga and Pilates can energise, strengthen and improve muscle tone. Plus, there's also an increasing number of sports-specific classes that would suit many men.

6 RESISTANCE TRAINING

Pushing weights is not the only way to overload muscles to increase their strength, size and power. Hill running, body weight moves, jumping exercises (plyometrics) and medicine ball work are all resistance training methods that can build stronger and more powerful muscle. From such a wealth of options you should be able to discover a method (or a combination of methods) that suits your training goals, your body type and your level of fitness.

When starting an exercise programme, regardless of body type it's crucial that you progress slowly and learn correct lifting technique.

However, I recommend that regardless of your fitness level or body type/shape you use free weights as opposed to fixed (machine) weights wherever possible. These are much more 'real world'. We don't lift or reach for objects within a cage that guides our limbs or torso, so why should we lift weights in a similar contrived fashion? There are some exceptions of course; for example, where a free weight exercise for a particular muscle group does not exist, as for the leg curl, or on occasions when lifting very heavy weights. In the latter case a Smith machine becomes a sensible option, but even these can compromise your body position and alter the dynamics of the exercise. Obviously a guy who is new to weight training should not load as much weight as possible on to a bar and then try to move it. I know it's

tempting, but don't do this if you don't want to look stupid or, worse still, injure yourself. Always, always underestimate what you think you can achieve when starting out on a weight training (or any other exercise) programme.

A word on weights belts: ditch them unless you have back problems or are a serious weight lifter. You need your core to interact with your limbs to stabilise your body when lifting. Get it strong through abdominal and back work and let it do the job. It will develop increased stabilising power in any case while weight training. To reiterate, always ensure that you have mastered the correct techniques for all the exercises you perform.

Selecting the 'right' weights exercises

There are thousands of weights (and resistance training) exercises from which to choose. Some work large muscle groups, such as the squat and the bench press (compound or multi-joint exercises), while others target smaller muscles such as the biceps curl (isolation or single joint exercises). The exercises you select and the weight training system you use will have a significant effect on how your body type responds to your workouts (see also training systems and hormonal response to weight training, page 22).

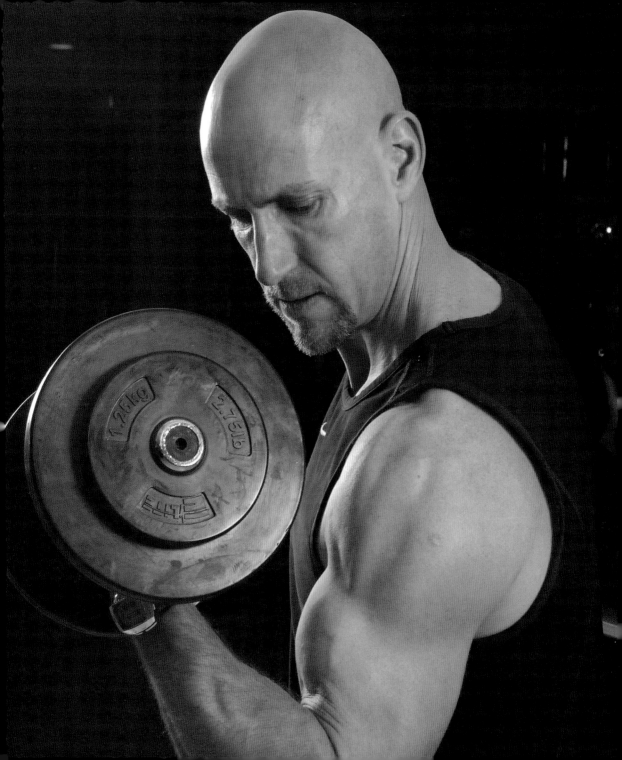

COMPOUND EXERCISES

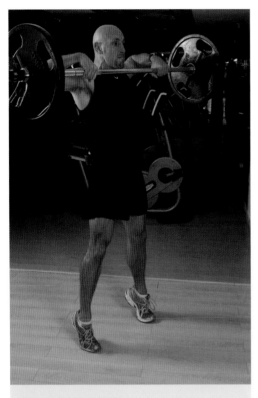

Fig. 6.1 *High pull*

Compound exercises work more than one large muscle group, across a number of joints – for example, the squat, clean or the high pull (which works the legs, torso and shoulders).

These exercises are very intense and are therefore great at eliciting an elevated anabolic hormone release (above that which could be expected from an isolation exercise, such as the biceps curl). With a greater dose of these hormones in your system your muscles will be primed to increase in size, strength and power.

For most body types compound exercises should be your bread and butter lifts if you are after increased lean muscle mass, reduced body fat, greater strength and power. For the really dynamic compound lifts, such as the high pull, snatch and clean, you must receive expert tuition and start with very light weights. For these lifts, technique is as important as brute strength. It is these lifts that have the greatest anabolic effect.

ISOLATION EXERCISES

Isolation exercises, such as the triceps extension, are best left to the end of your workout regardless of your body type, as they do not require as much energy to complete as compound exercises. You'll have more energy to get the 'big' ones out of the way at the start of your workout. End your workout with the isolation ones and your abdominal and back routines. (Note: If doing CV in your workouts, do this after your weights.)

Isolation exercises can be crucial for pre-conditioning purposes and avoiding injury for all body types.

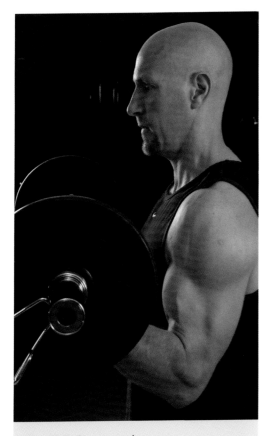

Fig. 6.2 *Biceps curl*

Training tip

Muscles are active tissue and require energy all day long just to sit on your body. For every 0.45kg gain, you could expect an additional 30–50 calories burn a day. That could be as many as 350 in a week – the equivalent of a 30-minute easy-pace run.

Therefore weights should be included in a training plan for weight loss. Because they will already be lean, ectomorphs will have to work harder to build more muscle. Diet and creating a positive calorie balance becomes crucial.

Knowing what to lift

The following guidelines will give you a good idea as to what's a 'heavy, medium and light' weight. I use these terms to reference the weight training workouts given later. The amount of weight you lift, plus the number of sets and repetitions, will have a significant effect on how your body adapts to the stimuli.

I have also indicated the intensity of the weights as a percentage of one repetition maximum (1RM). This refers to the maximum amount you could lift once on any one exercise. However, those new to weight training should not attempt to find their 1RMs and experienced trainers should establish new RMs regularly as

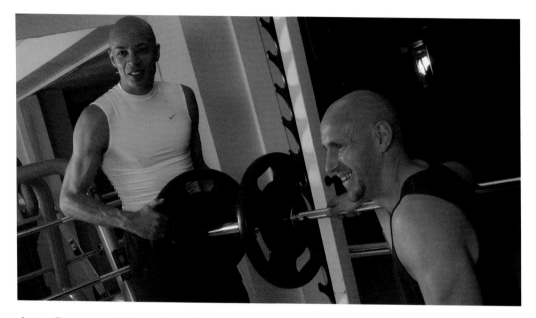

they will go up and down depending on your condition and time in the training year.

- Light weight (LW) – less than 65 per cent 1RM – approximates to a weight you could lift 10–30 times before fatigue sets in.
- Medium weight (MW) – 65–75 per cent 1RM – approximates to a weight you could lift 7–10 times before fatigue sets in.
- Medium heavy/heavy weight (MH/HW) – 75–85 per cent 1RM – approximates to a weight you could lift 5–7 times before fatigue sets in.
- Heavy weight (HW) – 85–100 per cent 1RM – approximates to a weight you could lift less than 5 times.

(Note: These are approximations – the number of repetitions you are actually able to perform will be governed by your current level of strength and fitness and even the exercise.)

Muscular action and strength development

It can be all too easy to complete a weights workout and not fully understand the effects it is having. You might be blissfully unaware

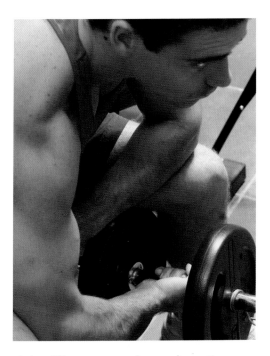

a biceps curl and running are examples of isotonic muscular actions.

- Concentric muscular action. A concentric contraction occurs when a muscle shortens as it contracts to create movement. It's the most common direction of effort for resistance and CV exercise. During a biceps curl, the biceps contract concentrically to raise the bar.
- Eccentric muscular action. An eccentric

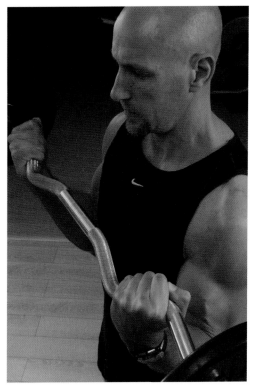

of the different types of muscular actions you can use to develop strength, power and size. I've identified specific 'strength types' below. They are suitable for all body types and shapes, as long as the individual is pre-conditioned, has mastered exercise technique, and is at the right stage in their training.

- Isotonic muscular action. Isotonic muscular action involves movement and incorporates 'concentric' and 'eccentric' actions. Curling and lowering a dumbbell when performing muscular action involves the lengthening of a muscle as it contracts to create movement. During a biceps curl, the biceps extend eccentrically to lower the bar and control the weight.

Research indicates that greater numbers of fast twitch, strength and power-increasing motor units and fibres are recruited when lifting eccentrically (see above). Thus eccentric training could be used by all body types looking to build more muscle. This is because it will hit the fibres that will hypertrophy (increase in size). You'll need a training partner or item of specially designed training kit to train eccentrically when lifting the medium-to-heavy and heavy weights necessary to stimulate muscle growth. The advanced weight trainer should be able to eccentrically lift super maximal loads up to 120 per cent of their concentric/eccentric 1RM.

Eccentric weight training is also referred to as negative repetition training (see Table 8).

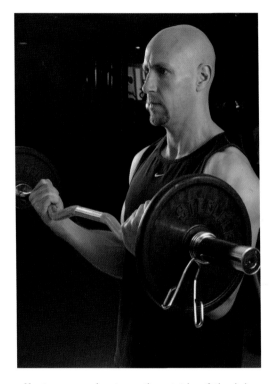

Isometric muscular action

During an isometric exercise no movement occurs. This is the result of opposing muscle groups working against each other, such as the biceps and triceps. Clasping your hands in front of your chest and pressing them together is an example of an isometric contraction. This type of training is not widely practised, as it is difficult to measure its overall effect on muscle strength outside of the laboratory. However, isometric muscle actions are involved in some way in nearly all everyday fitness and sports activities. For example, when performing a seated dumbbell shoulder press the muscles of the core (abdominal and back muscles) work isometrically to hold the trunk in position.

Isokinetic muscular action

Isokinetic muscular action involves moving a pre-set resistance (concentrically and/or eccentrically) over a full or part range of movement. Isokinetic resistance training machines exist in some gyms, although the majority of fixed weight installations are isotonic. Isokinetic machines are often used for injury rehabilitation purposes. Because of the constant resistance offered it is argued that they recruit more muscle fibre. Isokinetic machines are not as suitable for sports training as they remove the accelerative ability that most sports movements require.

By varying the type of muscular action involved you can continually stimulate your muscles (and mind), creating the optimum conditions needed for adaptation and avoiding training stagnation.

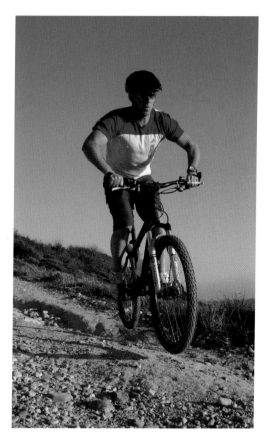

> ## Training tip
>
> **Train your brain as well as your muscles**
> Resistance training targets the nervous system as well as the muscles. In fact, it's estimated that as much as 20 per cent of the 'strength' required to perform a common weight training move, like the bench press, results from nervous activity. In time, an exercise becomes so 'patterned' into our brain (and consequentially our muscles) that less effort is required to complete it. This will slow training progression as the neuro-muscular system puts in less effort to do the job. This is why, as I stress many times throughout this book, you must constantly change, progress, adapt and cycle your training to optimise training progression (*see* 73).

Training tip

The power of suggestion

Tell yourself that you are getting stronger and that your training is working to change your body shape or make you a better sports player. Research indicates that those with a positive training outlook and belief in what they are doing will get greater results than those who don't. Some research has even found that concerted thinking about getting stronger will make you stronger!

Developing different types of strength

There are three main types of strength that can be developed through weight training – 'maximum', 'power' and 'endurance strength'. Each is determined by the percentage of 1RM that you work out at, the speed at which you move the weights, the recovery used, and the number of repetitions completed. This applies whatever your body type. You should develop the type of strength needed for your body type/shape, training goals, and level of fitness and any sports training goals you may have.

SOME BODY TYPES ARE BETTER SUITED TO LIFTING HEAVIER WEIGHTS

Endomorphs should find it easier to lift heavier weights due to their natural propensity for strength and greater muscle mass compared to ectomorphs, for example. Their muscles will also adapt more quickly in comparison.

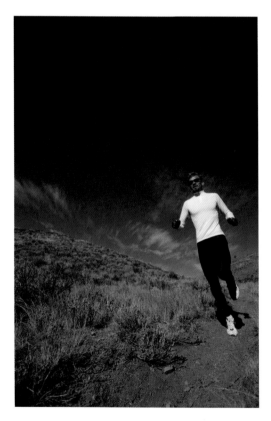

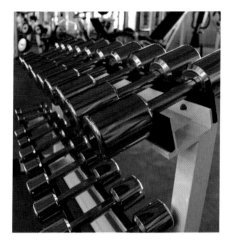

Training tip

You should work out with a training partner when maximum strength weight training. It's this person's job to 'spot' for you – that is, assist you to return the bar back to its starting position if you cannot complete your repetitions. Your training partner's presence and words of encouragement will also motivate you.

MAXIMUM STRENGTH WEIGHT TRAINING

Develops
The ability to lift very heavy weights.

Targets
Fast twitch muscle fibre, and has a moderate effect on increasing muscle size.

If you are after an increase in your absolute strength and muscle size, then using low repetitions (1 to 5) with heavy weights (85 per cent plus of 1RM) is the way to go. Recovery should be relatively long (2 to 5 minutes between sets) to maintain quality and intensity. Training for maximum strength is very draining. Correct technique (as for all weight training) is a must.

This type of training is particularly suited to endomorphs or those with endomorphic tendencies due to their natural strength.

Note that if you are new to weight training you should not do maximum strength weight training until you have developed a suitable foundation of strength at lower intensities.

Sample workouts
a) 4 x 3 @ 90% 1RM
b) 3 x 5 @ 80% 1RM
c) 8 x 1 @ 95% 1RM
Number of exercises: 4–6
Preferable exercise type: compound

POWER WEIGHT TRAINING

Develops
The ability of the muscles and body to perform dynamic and powerful lifts and movements.

Targets

Fast twitch muscle fibre, and has a potentially large effect on increasing muscle size (due to hormonal response) – particularly suited to sports training and body building.

Power weight training is very intense. It uses medium to medium/heavy weights – 65–85 per cent of 1RM loadings, over 5 to 10 repetitions and 3 to 6 sets. It differs from maximum strength weight training in that it requires dynamic, fast, but controlled lifting. As I've indicated, this type of lifting results in the greatest positive anabolic hormone release, making it suitable for all body types wanting increased muscle mass.

Recovery can vary between insufficient (less than a minute between sets) and sufficient (two to three minutes). With less recovery, research has indicated that the hormonal response may be even greater. (Note: This method is not suitable for those new to weight training, regardless of body type.)

Sample workouts

a) 3 x 8 @ 70% 1RM – number of exercises: 6
b) 4 x 4 @ 80% 1RM – number of exercises: 4

Training tip

Power weight training develops a foundation of specific strength for those involved in sports such as football, tennis and track and field.

Preferable exercise type: compound and dynamic compound, such as cleans and high pulls.

STRENGTH ENDURANCE WEIGHT TRAINING

Develops

Muscles' ability to continue to contract under conditions of fatigue and will tone.

Targets

Slow twitch muscle fibre, and has little effect on increasing muscle size.

Weight training develops strength endurance when high numbers of repetitions (10–30) are combined with light weights (30–60 per cent of 1RM) and short recoveries. This type of workout can be particularly useful for mesomorphs and endomorphs who want to lose weight. This is because these workouts can have a significant aerobic effect and will complement any CV work that is being performed – due to greater energy system synergy.

Sample workout

4 x 20 @ 50% 1RM

Number of exercises: 6–15 (select exercises for all body parts. Recovery, 30 seconds or less between sets).

Preferable exercise type: both isolation and compound (can also include body weight and plyometric exercises).

Keep changing your routines to get the most from your weight training

It's all too easy to do the same workout over and over again. We could be in and out of the gym before we know it with our brains on autopilot. This will diminish the opportunity for continued muscular development, due to a lack of mental and physical stimulation. To prevent this, the emphasis of our workouts should be changed every 6–8 weeks. This can be achieved, for example, by switching from different weight training systems, altering the type of strength being trained for and varying exercise selection.

Don't perform the same number of repetitions for every exercise in your workout

In the same way that we can be on 'workout autopilot', we'll very often complete workouts that use the same number of repetitions across all exercises – for example, 3 x 8 repetitions at 75 per cent 1RM on squat, bench press, clean and lunge. A team of researchers from Connecticut set out to discover whether doing this was indeed the most effective way of

increasing strength. Their study[vi] involved trained and untrained men. Specifically they wanted to determine what the maximal number of repetitions were that the two groups could perform doing free weight exercises at various percentages of 1RM. Eight trained and eight untrained men were tested for 1RM strength; they then performed 1 set to failure at 60, 80, and 90 per cent of 1RM in the back squat, bench press and arm curl.

The team discovered that more back squat repetitions could be performed than bench presses or arm curls at 60, 80 and 90 per cent 1RM by both groups (although this was less pronounced at the higher 1RM percentages). The team concluded that the number of repetitions performed at a given percentage of 1RM is influenced by the amount of muscle mass used during the exercise, as more repetitions can be performed during the back squat than either the bench press or arm curl. Also, they concluded that the training status of the individual has a minimal impact on the number of repetitions performed at relative exercise intensities. The implications for guys looking to increase strength are fairly obvious in this respect; the number of repetitions employed at all percentages of 1RM should reflect the amount of muscle mass recruited by the exercise – that is, the greater the muscle mass recruited, the more repetitions you should complete. Doing this should maximise the training effect.

[vi] *J Strength Cond Res*, 2006, Nov; 20(4): 819–23.

Training tip

Achieving a 'cut' physique

OK, you're in the gym training. Take a look at the guys around you and consider the body shapes, body types and the 'look' of your fellow weight trainers. You might see two guys with very similar body types, but quite different 'looks'. This is often the case with the permutations of mesomorphs. There will be guys training for muscle size (perhaps, using very heavy weights) and those for power (moving medium-weight weights quickly, for example), maybe because they need it for their sport. Look closely and you'll see that the latter mesomorph will invariably have less body fat and look leaner, less bulky and more athletic than the strength-training mesomorph. This is largely a consequence of 1) their more varied training regime; they'll probably be performing anaerobic and aerobic workouts and plyometrics with the resultant greater calorie burn, and 2) the fact that their workout programme stimulates a greater release of the anabolic and fat-burning hormones, testosterone and growth hormone.

Complement your weight training with other resistance training methods

To achieve a leaner, more defined muscled physique I recommend that you complement your weight training with other resistance training, such as body weight exercises, plyometrics and/or sports training. This additional training can increase muscle definition and boost metabolic rate. It will also make your workouts more varied and therefore more stimulating.

Weight training and sports involvement

Note that muscle weighs more than other body tissue and so, in sports where power to weight ratio is important (e.g. long jumping), putting on too much muscle can actually be counterproductive. These athletes and their coaches must tread a careful path and carefully consider the anabolic effects of weight workouts.

Weight training systems

There are hundreds of weight training systems from which to choose. A weight training system combines different combinations of sets and repetitions and the amount of weight used to overload muscles. Pyramids are a well-known example, where the weight is usually increased as the numbers of reps are decreased as sets are progressed.

As with the ways that you can develop different types of strength through weight training, it is important to consider the effects that different weight training systems can have on your body type/shape (*see* Table 8).

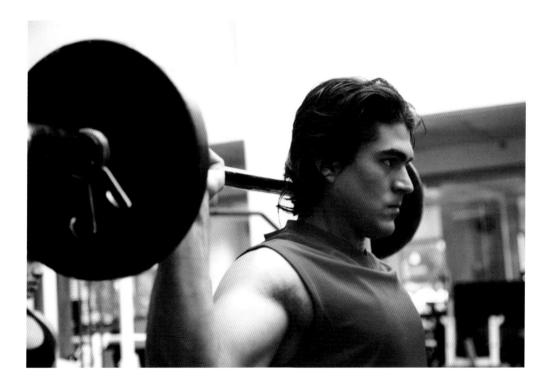

Overview of the effects of selected weight training systems on body type/shape

SIMPLE SETS

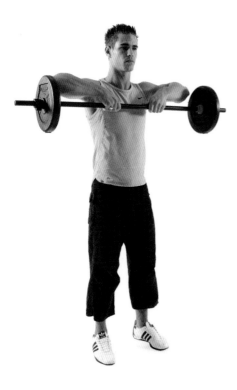

Description

Combines usually the same number of reps, e.g. 10 with a designated number of sets.
Example: 4 x 10.

Note: Recent research has highlighted the need to use greater numbers of reps for compound exercises as opposed to isolation exercises (*see* page 64)

Effect on selected body type

Largely depends on the amount of weight lifted (*see* 'Developing different types of strength', page 70). Ectomorphs wanting larger muscles are best advised to avoid light-weight, high-rep simple sets as these could actually reduce muscle mass by increasing metabolic rate and not stimulating muscle growth.

Comments

Despite their name, simple sets are a very effective form of training – suitable for all levels of fitness. Vary the weight lifted, the number of reps and recovery to create different training effects.

DROP SETS

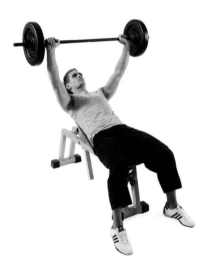

Effect on selected body type

This system will have a serious anabolic effect and significantly overload muscles (all fibre types). As such, it is a good option for the meso-morph or endomorph looking for increased muscle size.

Comments

This is an advanced system and should only be used by the experienced weight trainer, and then very selectively. At least 48 hours' recovery must be taken after such workouts. Protein consumption should begin immediately after-wards (*see* page 137).

Description

This intense method of training begins with a heavy load on the bar, and as many reps as possible are completed. Weight is then taken off the bar and as many reps as possible are completed again. This process continues for a designated number of sets or until there is no weight left on the bar!

SUPER-SETS

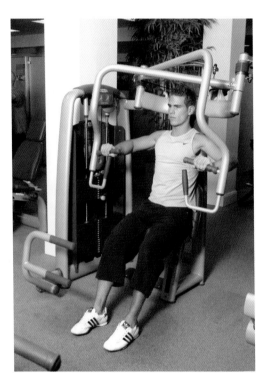

Description

Super-sets contain pairings (or more) of exercises that usually target the same muscle/muscle group (e.g. bench press and chest flyes for the pectorals). They can also work opposing muscle groups, such as the biceps and triceps, with biceps curls and triceps curls. One set is performed of one exercise, then the other immediately afterwards. A short recovery can be taken and then the next set is performed.

Effect on selected body type

Super-sets are great for hitting muscle fibre and stimulating growth, particularly if they target the same muscle group and medium to heavy weights are used.

Comments

Suitable for intermediate and advanced weight trainers.

COMPLEX TRAINING

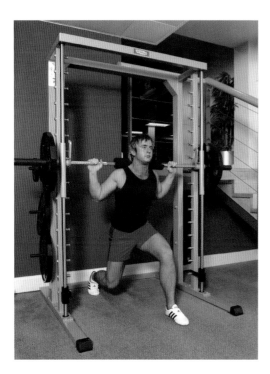

Description
A type of super-sets can also be performed with a mix of weight training and plyometric exercises that work the same muscle groups (e.g. the squat and squat jumps), which is also known as complex training. Such training is great for boosting sports performance as it hits fast twitch muscle fibres hard.

Effect on selected body type
Will increase muscular power output.

Comments
Not suitable for those new to resistance training. Pre-conditioning is a must before performing such a dynamic training system.

PRE-EXHAUST, POST-PUMP

Description
An isolation move that targets a muscle involved in a compound move is performed before the compound move; for example, the triceps kick back before the bench press.

Effect on selected body type
The first exercise reduces the targeted muscle's potential contribution to the latter. This means that the major muscles involved in the compound exercise receive a greater emphasis, as does the muscle involved in the isolation exercise.

Comments
Suitable for advanced weight trainers only, as the dynamics of the exercise can be affected by the prior performance of the isolation move. As with drop sets, this system should be used sparingly.

SPLIT ROUTINE

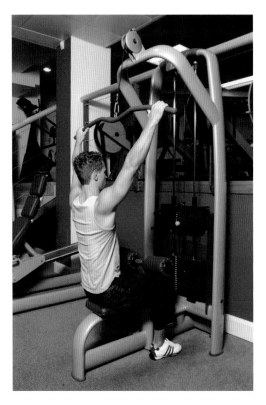

Effect on selected body type

Ectomophs (and any body type after increased muscle size) can benefit from this system. This is because maximum mental and physical effort can be put into the training of each body region and because the system allows for relatively long periods of muscle growing recovery between workouts.

Comments

Suitable for intermediate and advanced trainers.

Description

Body regions, such as the legs, chest and shoulders, are exercised over separate workouts. This enables maximum effort to be put into the relevant weights exercises during each split routine workout.

NEGATIVE (ECCENTRIC LIFTS)

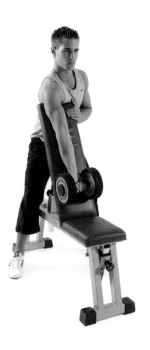

Effect on selected body type
Can be used by all body types wanting increased size and strength.

Comments
Suitable for intermediate and advanced trainers. Note: A training partner will normally be required, to assist the return of the weights to the starting position before the next rep can be completed. (*See* the *Complete Guide to Sports Training* by John Shepherd, A&C Black, 2006.)

Description
These workouts emphasise the lowering (eccentric muscular contraction) phase of the lift. Take a slow 5–8 count as you lower the weight. Note super maximum weights (100–120% of 1RM) will achieve the best results.

FORCED REPS

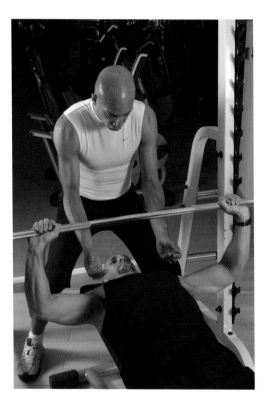

Description

With the aid of a training partner you 'force' out 1 or 2 additional reps when you would not normally be able to do so at the end of your sets.

Effect on selected body type

Suitable for all body types.

Comments

Advanced training option. Requires considerable neural input. Should be used sparingly – but is a possible way to break through a weight training plateau. Take 48 hours' recovery after these workouts to maximise muscle growth.

The importance of the last rep – the 'growth' rep

In order to develop maximum strength and strength endurance and create the 'right' conditions in your muscles for growth, the last rep should be difficult to perform. This will force your muscles into unknown territory and break down muscle protein that will be re-built during non-training time, resulting in stronger (and potentially larger) muscle fibres. If you fail to do this regularly, then your strength and muscle development will not progress as much as you would probably want it to.

Maintain good technique

Despite the effort you need to put in to complete the last rep, you must do this without loss of good technique. Power weight training is slightly different in this respect as it is the speed of lift that matters. As such, performing slower reps with poor technique due to fatigue is counter-productive. It is better to cut back on your reps or take a greater recovery during a workout if fatigue begins to impair your performance.

Keep your weight training gains coming

MUSCULAR ADAPTATION
Contrary to much 'gym wisdom', muscles grow when you are *not* training. After a weights

workout, muscle protein that has been broken down needs to be re-synthesised and repaired. Rest (see below) and optimum nutrition (see part 3) are crucial for this to happen. Although this applies to all body types, advanced weight training mesomorphs can get away with less recovery, but if they do this they may become over-trained. Signs of over-training include tiredness, aching muscles and a lack of

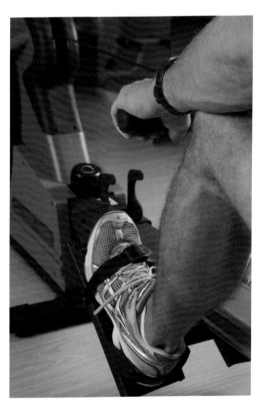

training motivation. All body types should schedule in adequate rest in their training plans and be aware of over-training symptoms.

For more information on over-training, *see* page 101.

REST

It can take up to 48 hours to recover fully from a weights workout. Sleep is particularly crucial as this is when growth hormone release is at its strongest and the repair and growth processes occur in your muscles. You should aim for 7–8 hours of sleep a day. To facilitate this, you should adopt a regular sleeping routine.

DON'T GET STUCK IN A TRAINING RUT

Workouts must be constantly progressed otherwise training gains will come to a halt. There are many ways of doing this:

- Vary the weight training system
- Vary the type of strength
- Use dumbbells instead of barbells.

HOW MUCH MUSCLE GAIN CAN YOU EXPECT?

The million dollar question! The answer: 0.5–1kg per month, perhaps more when you start a weight training programme designed to achieve greater size. Supplementing with crea-

tine could also give your muscle building a boost. Many men report significant lean muscle gains with its use (*see* page 128).

Note that you will reach a limit as the training years progress; and, as you age, it becomes more a matter of maintenance.

Shaping the male physique – resistance training

With the right weight (other resistance and CV) training we can shape our bodies to maximise the way we look. However, we'll need to carefully select the appropriate exercises, weight training system and the type of strength we want to develop, and couple all this to a systematic training and optimum nutrition plan. Doing this will provide every opportunity of adjusting our proportions. It may take time, but the journey is well worth it. Here are some tips:

CONCENTRATE ON THE MUSCLES YOU CAN'T SEE AS WELL AS THOSE YOU CAN SEE

Many guys 'forget' about the muscles that they can't see, such as those to the back of their body. This over-emphasis on bench pressing, for example, can result in a pigeon-chested look. You need to 'balance' your body, and to do this you need to analyse its proportions and select the appropriate exercises for you. I have provided some examples as to how certain weight training exercises can 'improve' your proportions.

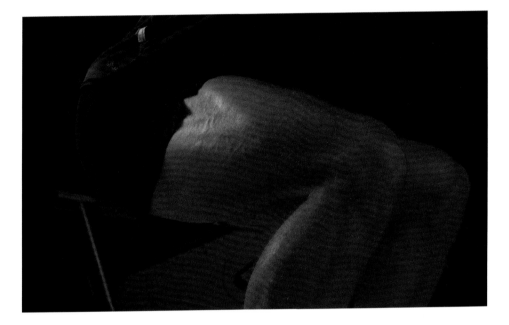

DON'T FORGET YOUR LEGS

Many guys who are 'into' getting bigger seemingly 'forget' to train their legs but go all out on their torsos. Training the legs is important for aesthetic reasons and also because of the amount of muscle that is recruited during lifts such as the squat. This will boost hormone response across the whole body, potentially leading to greater leanness, thus improving overall appearance.

Training tip

Some men perform endless biceps curls in an attempt to make this muscle more visible. However, training the triceps could be just as profitable, if not more. This is because this muscle is about a third bigger than the biceps, and thus when trained appropriately can add greater size to the upper arms.

USING WEIGHTS TO REDUCE YOUR PROPORTIONS

If you are an endomorph and/or overweight, then weight training can help you reduce your non-lean fat weight and assist your quest for a more aesthetic shape. It will achieve this in two ways:

1 The addition of more lean muscle to your body will enhance your metabolic rate. As noted, muscle is metabolically active tissue and burns calories at rest.
2 Weight training has a significant effect on post-workout calorie burning (*see* page 88).

Strength endurance weight training is a particularly suitable method of weight training for weight loss, as it has a significant CV calorie-burning effect and EPOC (*see* page 54). You will also profit most from an X-training programme that combines CV work with weights (and other training options).

CYCLE YOUR TRAINING

You've been training for size, for example, for a couple of months, and now is the time to switch and train for power or strength endurance for 6–8 weeks. Doing this will keep your mind and your muscles stimulated. No athlete performs the same type of training all year round; rather, he alternates and gradually adapts his training to bring about peak performance. You should do the same and follow what is known as a 'periodised' training plan (*see* page 88 for more information on how to plan your training for your body type).

Training tip

When using weights to shape your body, take a good look at your shape and match this against your body type. By doing this you'll know what routines are most likely to work for you and what areas to work on. Then select the most appropriate weights, exercises and systems to build the strength and shape you desire.

Training tip

Training the abdominals – the elusive six-pack

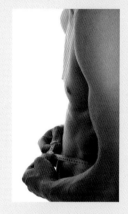

Obtaining a six-pack is one of the most sought after physical qualities among men. It can be incredibly difficult to actually achieve one, no matter your body type or how fit you are. And I know because I've tried. For the lucky few it can be more a case of genetics than anything else. In this respect, ecto-mesomorphs might be at a slight advantage as they will be carrying less body fat (which will not cover their abs) and have a body type that accumulates muscle relatively easily.

Paradoxically, achieving a six-pack is more about not training your abs than training them. You'll not get one by performing hundreds of sit-ups and crunches day in, day out, despite what you may think. Yes, you do need to do these exercises, but achieving a six-pack will be the result of a balanced training and nutrition programme. Think about it, your abs (and back muscles) are used in countless weight training, fitness, sports and everyday activities. They'll get a good workout during a set of press-ups or when performing seated overhead shoulder presses. Getting them 'on show' is more about diet and balancing CV training with your weight training than performing crunches.

However, I would like to advise the following when it comes to abdominal exercises in the pursuit of a six-pack – perform the exercises super slow and, for advanced trainers, with added resistance. Really focus on initiating the movement with your abs, so that you overload them. Lift and lower to a slow 'four' count. You'll soon feel the 'burn' even if you can knock out hundreds of faster-paced efforts. The slow concentric/eccentric muscular actions will engage more muscle fibre and prevent gravity and momentum reducing the effectiveness of your ab training.

POST-WORKOUT CALORIE-BURNING AND RESISTANCE TRAINING

In the previous CV section I pointed out how your body can continue to burn calories after your workout due to excess post-oxygen consumption (EPOC – *see* page 54) interestingly, this phenomenon also applies to resistance training.

Research indicates – as I have stressed throughout this book – that intensity is again the key to the magnitude of the effect when it comes to resistance training. The harder your session, for example, the more sets you perform, the greater your calorific burn will be when you put your feet up. As with CV trainers, post-workout calorie burning should be factored into your energy balance calculations regardless of your body type. Once you have been training regularly – three to four times a week – for a couple of months you should add 20 per cent on to your daily calorific needs, while still adding the calories expended for your workouts to provide you with a figure for your total daily needs (*see* pages 24 and 138 for a guide to calculating your calorific needs).

Table 8 Sample weight training plans for selected body types and training goals

Body type	Training experience	Training goals	Suggested workouts	Comment
Ectomorph	Intermediate	To gain lean muscle and maintain general health	1) Super-sets for chest and legs using medium to heavy weights – compound exercises 2) Simple sets – power, weight strength type, medium weights, using compound exercises 3) Eccentric workout using medium to heavy weights – compound exercises	These weights workouts are designed to optimise hormonal response and target fast-twitch muscle fibre

Body type	Training experience	Training goals	Suggested workouts	Comment
Endomorph	Intermediate	To lose weight	1) Strength endurance, simple set workout using light weights, compound and single joint exercises 2) Simple set workout using medium weights, compound and single joint exercises 3) Body weight circuit (or boxing-based class)	The aim is to rev up metabolic rate and add to the achievement of a negative energy balance. Do alongside CV workouts. Lean muscle mass also boosts everyday calorie burning (complete 2–3 sessions of CV work per week – *see* page 45)
Mesomorph	Advanced	Significant increase in muscle mass	1) Simple sets in high numbers (8–10) and reps (8–10) using power training methodology, compound and single joint exercises 2) and 3). Split routine for chest, back, legs, abs and shoulders, using heavy weights (maximum strength type) compound exercises. Could also include forced reps (page 82).	This is a very tough regime that shocks muscles into growth. It requires considerable mental input, and should be stringently monitored to prevent over-training and used sparingly.

Table 8 Sample weight training plans for selected body types and training goals (cont.)

Muscle memory

Research indicates that previously trained muscle will regain strength more quickly than the untrained muscle. This means that those returning to weight training will gain strength more rapidly than those embarking on a training programme for the first time.

De-training

When you stop training, your muscle strength and mass will gradually decline, and these changes will become noticeable after 2–3 weeks of inactivity. Interestingly, if your muscles seem to become bigger after a week and you return to the gym stronger than before you left, the chances are that you were previously over-training. This will also result from the tapering of your training and the coming to a peak.

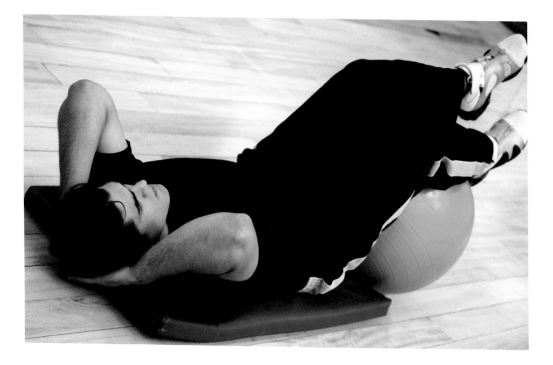

7 SPORTS TRAINING AND BODY TYPE

Many men play sport. In this brief section I identify how your body type can affect your sports choice and identify some training issues.

Body type can have a big influence on the sports that seem suited to you. For example, endomorphs will make potentially good rugby forwards or shot putters. Mesomorphs will be suited to most sports, and ectomorphs to endurance activities. However, there will always be exceptions, and your desire to want to play a particular sport is crucial in this respect, as is following a relevant training programme. I indicated in Part 1 that nurture and your genetic make-up are also powerful influences on how your body will adapt to training as well as body type. Although there do seem to be certain 'typical' characteristics of players in certain sports, and even positions, these can be challenged.

Power training, sports performance and body type

Power is a vital commodity for sport's performance and is very closely associated with speed with regard to its development. Your body type – as it affects your strength and CV capability – will also have a strong influence on your ability to express power. Mesomorphs and endomorphs will have greater muscle mass and the capability to achieve greater levels of mass. This can be beneficial as, every-thing else being equal, a larger muscle offers greater potential power output. However, these larger muscles must be 'made' to express power. If this were not the case, then

> ### Training tip
>
> You might have a mesomorphic/endomorphic body type, perhaps you are a long jump athlete or basketball player. You find that your body responds well to weight training and builds muscle. However, your sport's performance could be negatively affected because of this, as a result of significant increases in body weight (due to muscle gain and its heavier weight than other body tissue). Selecting the 'right' weights programme in terms of hormonal response could keep your muscles strong and powerful, yet smaller and with less of an effect on your weight. Your 'power to weight ratio' is crucial. To this end you may profit from heavy weight, maximum strength-developing training as noted previously, using low reps, as opposed to power weight sessions with medium to heavy weights and multiple reps and sets. This is because the former method will not have such a significant hormonal effect in terms of increasing muscle size (and therefore body weight) than the latter.

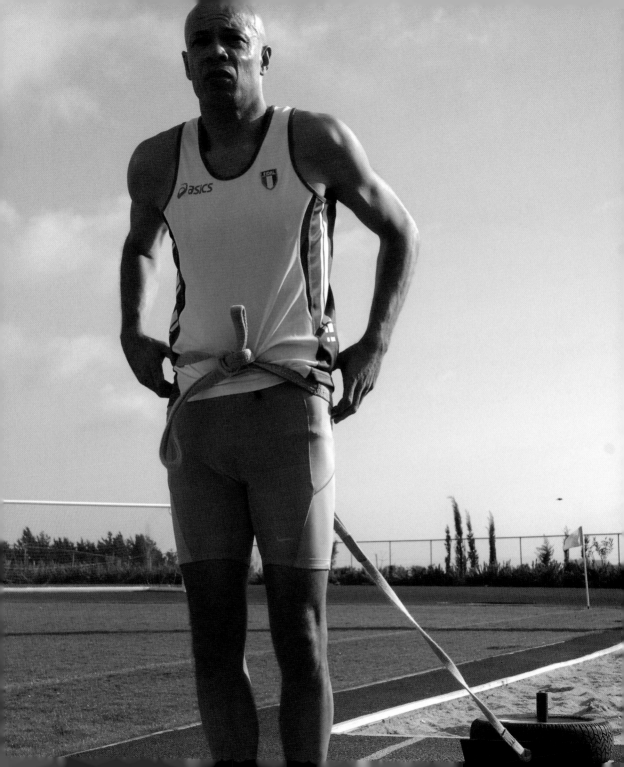

bodybuilders, with their huge muscles, would also be the fastest sprinters. Whatever your body type, you need to perform relevant exercise that will develop fast, reactive and dynamic muscle if you desire sports power.

Examples of relevant sports dynamic warm-up methods are found on pages 33–7.

Plyometric training

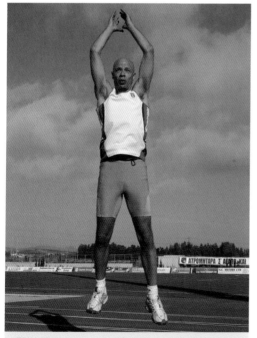

Fig. 7.1 *Keep your landing light to maximise the plyometric effect*

Plyometric training is perhaps the key training weapon in the sports training armoury. Such exercises utilise a unique muscular capability known as the 'stretch reflex'. This occurs when a concentric muscle contraction immediately follows a concentric one. This happens, for example, when jumping. It's a bit like stretching a spring to its fullest length (the eccentric contraction) and then releasing it (the concentric contraction). Immense amounts of energy will be released as the spring recoils.

See page 20 for more information on types of muscle contraction.

To train your muscles plyometrically you need to perform dynamic exercises, such as hops, bounds, jump squats, split jumps and jump (plyo) press-ups.

PLYOMETRIC TRAINING AND BODY TYPE TRAINING TIPS

Endomorphs
If you are an endomorph (or overweight), high-intensity plyometric exercises (such as hopping) are best avoided due to the loading placed on the ankles, knees and back, which could lead to injury. However, this does not mean that you cannot incorporate plyometrics into your training; rather, you need to select exercises that place less strain on your joints and progress gradually. In this respect, exercises

performed on the spot and involving double leg landings, such as jump squats, would be suitable.

Mesomorphs

Mesomorphs will be able to perform most plyometric exercises and will often be fast movers. However, if they have endomorphic tendencies, then they too will need to moderate plyometric usage and perhaps embark on an additional training programme and dietary regime to moderate their weight. Nor should they (like all body types) forget the value of pre-conditioning to avoid injury.

Ectomorphs

Ectomorphs will need to pre-condition to prepare their bodies for plyometric training – a period of focused weight and resistance exercises on the ankles, knees and core, and a gradual progression to more intense forms of plyometric exercises, such as hops, should be followed. However, their light frames can make them particularly powerful and create a very explosive power to weight ratio. As the percentages of fast and slow twitch muscle fibres are relatively evenly distributed among men (45–55 per cent fast twitch; 45–55 per cent slow twitch), it is possible that with the 'right' training ectomorphs can excel in certain sports that might usually be seen as more suited to bigger guys. My own sport of long

jump comes to mind here. With a light body and powerful muscles, the capabilities for long jumps become quite apparent. There is more of an issue in field sports where the power capability of the relevantly trained ectomorph can be compromised by their slim frame. This can make them more vulnerable to being 'muscled' off of the ball, for example, if playing football.

> **Training tip**
>
> Regardless of your body type, you must always pre-condition to avoid injury if you are a serious sports trainer.

> **Training tip**
>
> The most important aspect of training for a sport, whatever your body type, is the specificity of the training you do for your chosen activity. You and your coach must analyse the movement patterns, endurance, speed and power required and train appropriately. Training must be specific and mirror, where possible, what happens in the competition arena.

8 TRAINING PLANNING AND THE MENTAL APPROACH

Regardless of your body type, you won't get the most from it unless you work out to a systematic and focused training plan. In this chapter I show you how to plan your workouts to achieve the greatest gains, whatever your goals.

Don't be afraid to ask for help

Being guys, we often want quick results. We may charge into the gym and do as much as we can without thought to 1) whether the workout is actually doing us any good, and 2) whether we might injure ourselves in the process. OK, it is good to be aggressive when training, but this needs to be harnessed, controlled and focused. Nor should we be afraid to ask for help; personal trainers and gym instructors are there to assist our training. Don't think you know it all. Often a well-informed, second pair of eyes will make all the

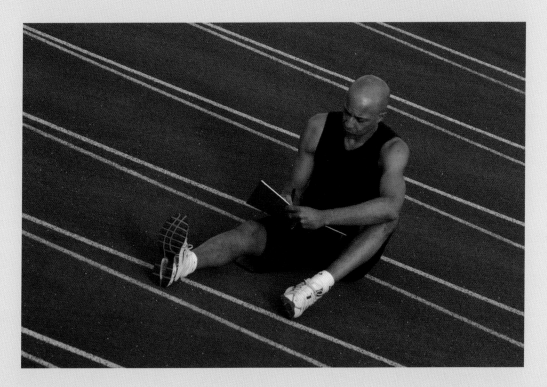

difference. Personal trainers and gym instructors can motivate and ensure that you work out safely and effectively. In our increasingly time-poor lives, they can offer a way to maximise our gym time, so that it is not wasted. A weekly session with a personal trainer can keep us focused and on course to reach our goals. They can monitor progress and tweak training so that we continue to improve. Even the most experienced trainer can still learn something.

Planning your training

If you intend to plan your own workouts, you should follow the steps I've provided. However, if you are new to training or are returning after a long lay-off, I would recommend that you book a couple of sessions with a personal trainer. I'd also recommend that you consult your GP, particularly if you are over 35.

Pulling it all together – constructing a training plan for your body type

STEP 1: ANALYSE YOUR BODY TYPE AND SHAPE

Using the information provided in this book, you should be able to determine your body type, current body shape and whether, for

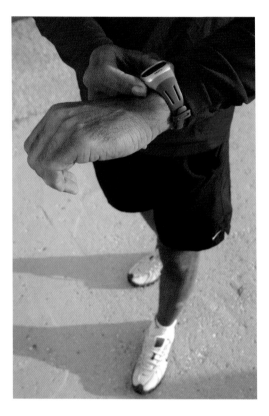

example, you need to lose or gain weight. For example, you may be a slightly overweight mesomorph, or an overweight endomorph and want to lose weight, or an ecto-mesomorph after weight gain. Once you have done this, you will be in a much more informed position to select the best training options for your body type and training goals.

STEP 2: SET SOME GOALS

Without goals you will not be able to line up your training. Goals are important motivators. You'll need short- and long-term ones. The former will act as stepping stones on the way to achieving the latter.

Use the SMART goal-setting principles. Your goals should be:

- Specific
- Measurable
- Achievable
- Realistic
- Targeted

Example:
Body shape: meso-endomorph, slightly over-weight (BMI score of 28 – see page 10)

Training goal: to reduce body fat and fall within acceptable BMI levels in four months

STEP 3: CONSTRUCTING YOUR TRAINING PLAN

A simple way to plan your training is to use the training pyramid concept. Basically, this model builds increased levels of fitness on previous levels of fitness as you progress to your goal – the apex of the pyramid. The training pyramid can be applied to any fitness (or sports training) goal. Each phase should be long enough (usually between 6 and 18 weeks) to allow your body to optimally adapt, without stagnation setting in or over-training. When planning your workouts you should allow a minimum of three months to reach the top of the pyramid and achieve your fitness goal/goals.

Note that mesomorphs may adapt more quickly to training and must continuously monitor their progress and adapt their training to avoid reduced training returns.

I have provided a basic training pyramid model that you can adapt to your own training goals and body type. It has three distinct training phases and one rest and recovery phase. You could design a pyramid with more training phases if you desired, if your training goal/goals were specific enough to warrant this. But for most general fitness purposes, three are sufficient. To make it easier for you to under-stand what to include in each phase, I've provided examples of potential workouts. I have designed it around a new-to-exercise overweight endomorph who wants to lose weight.

See also progressive overload (page 100) for a guide to how to progress your training.

Body type: endomorph
Fitness level: new to exercise
SMART training goal: to achieve acceptable BMI score (20–25, see page 10) and add shape to torso in 4 months

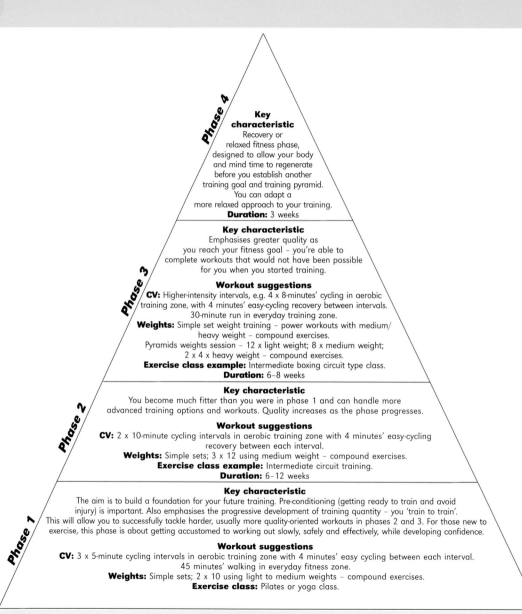

Phase 4

Key characteristic
Recovery or
relaxed fitness phase,
designed to allow your body
and mind time to regenerate
before you establish another
training goal and training pyramid.
You can adapt a
more relaxed approach to your training.
Duration: 3 weeks

Phase 3

Key characteristic
Emphasises greater quality as
you reach your fitness goal – you're able to
complete workouts that would not have been possible
for you when you started training.

Workout suggestions
CV: Higher-intensity intervals, e.g. 4 x 8-minutes' cycling in aerobic
training zone, with 4 minutes' easy-cycling recovery between intervals.
30-minute run in everyday training zone.
Weights: Simple set weight training – power workouts with medium/
heavy weight – compound exercises.
Pyramids weights session – 12 x light weight; 8 x medium weight;
2 x 4 x heavy weight – compound exercises.
Exercise class example: Intermediate boxing circuit type class.
Duration: 6–8 weeks

Phase 2

Key characteristic
You become much fitter than you were in phase 1 and can handle more
advanced training options and workouts. Quality increases as the phase progresses.

Workout suggestions
CV: 2 x 10-minute cycling intervals in aerobic training zone with 4 minutes' easy-cycling
recovery between each interval.
Weights: Simple sets; 3 x 12 using medium weight – compound exercises.
Exercise class example: Intermediate circuit training.
Duration: 6–12 weeks

Phase 1

Key characteristic
The aim is to build a foundation for your future training. Pre-conditioning (getting ready to train and avoid
injury) is important. Also emphasises the progressive development of training quantity – you 'train to train'.
This will allow you to successfully tackle harder, usually more quality-oriented workouts in phases 2 and 3. For those new to
exercise, this phase is about getting accustomed to working out slowly, safely and effectively, while developing confidence.

Workout suggestions
CV: 3 x 5-minute cycling intervals in aerobic training zone with 4 minutes' easy cycling between each interval.
45 minutes' walking in everyday fitness zone.
Weights: Simple sets; 2 x 10 using light to medium weights – compound exercises.
Exercise class: Pilates or yoga class.

Fig. 8.1 *The training pyramid*

Exercises to work the chest, shoulders and back should be selected for the torso. The 'endomorph' will respond well to training and develop muscle. Noticeable results should accrue from the end of phase 1. It is important to balance exercise selection. To give shape to the torso, more shoulder and back exercises may be needed to reduce the potential barrel shape that may develop from an over-emphasis on the chest. Suitable exercises would therefore include lat pull downs, lateral dumbbell shoulder lifts, and single and seated rows.

(Note: It is beyond the scope of this book to cover all the potential weights exercises or types of CV workouts that could be chosen, for this or other training goals. The key is to continually progress and vary the intensities of your workouts to effect the changes you desire. If unsure, you should ask your gym instructor or personal trainer to provide you with other relevant exercise possibilities and training options.)

Training tip

To get the most from your training you need to adopt a cyclical approach, emphasising various training aspects, components and variables at different times to achieve progressive and optimum results. The training pyramid is ideal in this respect.

The training variables

The variables of quantity, quality, duration, intensity and rest are fundamental to constructing a progressive training plan – they will inform and shape your individual workouts and overall plan.

- Quantity refers to the amount of training done either in a particular workout or as part of a particular training phase. It can be measured by the number of kilometres covered for CV training, or total weight lifted, repetitions or sets completed for weight training.
- Quality usually reflects the intensity of a workout. A low-quality workout may involve an easy-pace run; a high-quality one (at a high percentage of HRMax) or a series of near flat-out intervals. You should balance the quality of your workouts over your training plan to avoid over-training and potential injury.
- Duration applies to the length of a workout and is therefore more applicable to CV training than weight training. In this respect, it references the length of a workout or particular aspect of it (such as an interval) and is inextricably linked to quantity and quality.
- Frequency refers to the number of weekly or other period workouts.

■ Rest is just as important as training – this is when all the benefits accrue. Without sufficient rest, adaptive processes will not take place. Rest days, rest periods and the carefully constructed use of light, medium and tough workouts are all crucial to the balanced training plan.

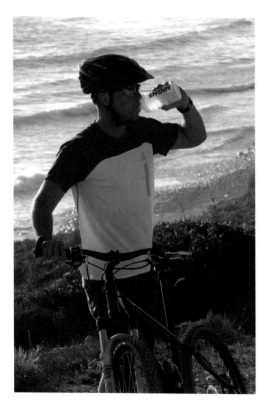

Progressive overload and adaptation

Progressive overload is one of the key principles of training. Put simply, if you don't progressively overload (lift heavier weights, perform more reps or run for further or faster, for example), you won't improve your fitness (adapt), whatever your body type.

Don't start off at a too intense level as this will lead to disappointment when you can't, for example, complete as many weights reps as you think you should, or, at worst, injury. Rather, begin at a low intensity and allow enough time between sessions for recovery. In time your body will adapt – you'll find lifting the weights easier. At this point you can then increase the intensity to produce further increases in fitness. If there is no progression, then your fitness level will plateau.

Table 9 Example of a progressive overload programme – particularly suited to those new to exercise				
Week	1 and 2	3 and 4	5 and 6	7 and 8
Reps and sets	2 sets x 5 reps	3 sets x 5 reps	3 sets x 8 reps	3 sets x 10 reps
Frequency	2 x per week	2 x per week	2 x per week	2 x per week

Table 9 shows a simple 'volume progression'. The goal at the start is to learn the exercises correctly. In this example, you perform only 2 sets x 5 reps twice a week for weeks 1 and 2, to ensure the muscles and tendons involved in the exercise are not overloaded too much too soon. During weeks 3 and 4 you complete 50 per cent more reps by adding another set (3 x 5). Over the next 4 weeks, you build up to 3 sets x 10 reps, which is three times the original quantity.

Over-training

Although exercise is good for you, there are times when too much of it can have a detrimental effect and potentially lead to over-training syndrome (OTS). A carefully constructed training programme incorporating sufficient rest and recovery should avoid OTS. But if you do suffer from some of the symptoms in the box opposite, and have been in hard training for a while, you could be suffering from OTS. If you think that you are, you should take at least a week off training before returning to your workouts, and then at a lower level than when you stopped. If you still suffer from the symptoms on your return to training, ease back for a further three weeks. If the symptoms quickly reappear when you eventually resume training, consult your doctor.

OVER-TRAINING SYMPTOMS

- A lack of desire to want to train.
- Continuously feeling fatigued and listless.
- Decreased maximal heart rate.
- Greater susceptibility to illness – particularly upper respiratory tract infections.
- Mood swings.
- Feelings of anxiousness and stress.
- An increase in resting heart rate.*
- Sleep problems.
- Lack of appetite.

*Resting heart rate (RHR) should be taken a few minutes after waking; an increase above 'normal' can indicate that you have not fully recovered from your previous workouts or are stressed. If your RHR has increased, then you should either take the day off from training or perform a light workout.

Training tip

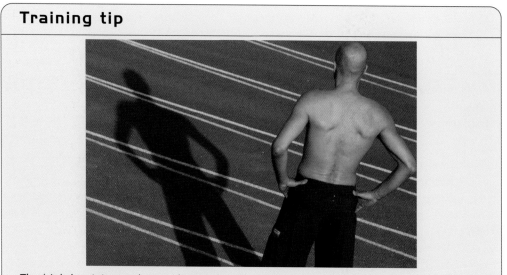

The 'right' training and mental attitude will get results.

I know that many guys are unhappy about their body shape, but are less inclined to admit it than women. In fact, a recent survey of 3000 men indicated that 1 in 4 felt uncomfortable getting undressed in front of their partners. So it is important to be positive and believe in the exercise and dietary regime that you are following, whatever your fitness or body shaping goals, if you want to make changes. It is equally important not to become disillusioned. A positive attitude could make all the difference. If you have established realistic training goals and an equally realistic training plan, then you will get results. Yes, certain body types will have to work harder than others to achieve their goals, but much is still possible.

Lifestyle – you can find the time to work out

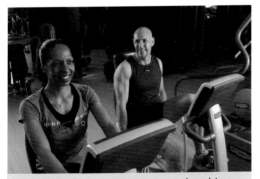

Fig. 8.2 *Get a joint gym membership for you and your partner and work out together*

Fitting in workouts and eating healthily can be a challenge, bearing in mind all the other constraints and distractions we have in our lives. However, there are many ways to do this.

Here are some really simple suggestions for fitting workouts into your daily routines: run or cycle to work, dust off the weights in the garage and use them, get a joint gym membership for you and your partner and work out together (that way, she can't say you're going there to get away from her), or take up an active weekend hobby like mountain biking. Or get yourself a rowing machine and sign up for a competition in six months' time. Any of these and other ideas will fit exercise into your lifestyle – in some cases, without you even realising it. You'll notice the difference physically and mentally as you acquire more energy and enjoy life much more.

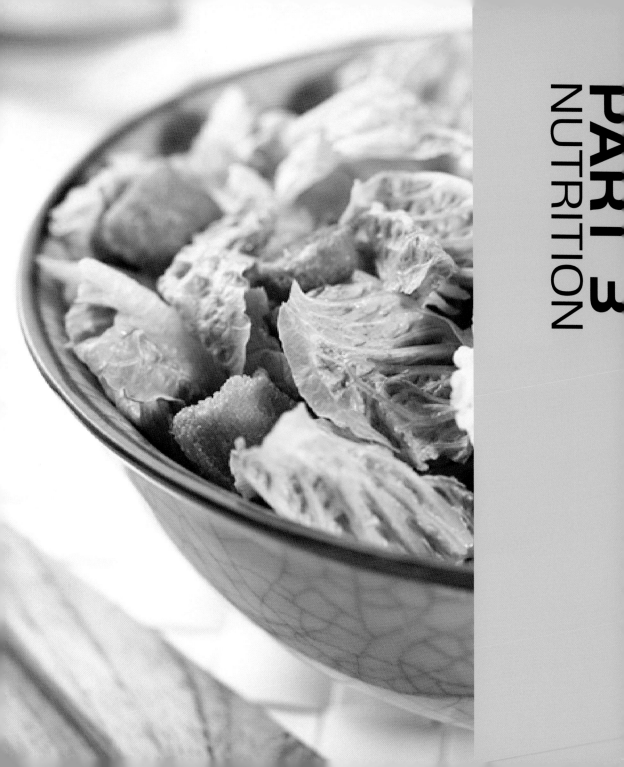

8

NUTRITION FOR YOUR BODY: THE BASICS, MACRO- AND MICRO-NUTRIENTS

Whatever your body type, how you fuel your body with food and drink is crucial to your health, fitness, body shaping and sports training goals. Each body type, depending on its training goals, will require a specific nutrition (and possibly supplement) plan. I will begin with an overview of the 'energy balance equation'. This will put into context your calorific and body type needs and indicate how much energy you will need to gain (lean weight), in order to maintain or lose weight. I then consider the main food groups (macro-nutrients) and explain what vitamins and minerals (micro-nutrients) and supplements can do for you. The calorie and macro-nutrient content of selected foods is then provided to make the process of food selection easier.

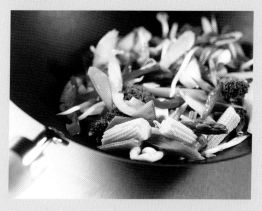

The information provided in this chapter should be read in conjunction with the practical training sections.

Food for life

As men, we may be less concerned about what we eat compared to women. Perhaps we are less 'educated' as to what's 'better' for us and what's not or maybe we're just lazy and live on a diet of fast food. Although information is much better than it used to be in terms of food labelling, healthy eating campaigns and numerous relevant TV shows, for example, it's obvious that this is not getting through to all

of us. If it were, then our levels of obesity would be declining rather than increasing.

Eating on the move and consuming convenience foods and takeaways will invariably result in you not getting the necessary vitamins and minerals needed for healthy bodily functioning and accumulating too much fat (*see* page 112). Like many guys, I was blissfully unaware of the huge potential that the micro-nutrients (vitamins and minerals) offered. It really does pay to buy the best food you can and to stop before you purchase a product or order from a menu and ask yourself, 'What good will that choice be for my body?' OK, it's just as unhealthy to become obsessive about what you eat, but we must be more concerned than ever, otherwise we will be less vital and positive about ourselves, and more likely to be ill and suffer from diseases.

And one final comment – designer or fad diets are best avoided. The best healthy eating programme is the one many of us will have been taught at school, with 60 per cent of our daily calories coming from carbohydrate (preferably unrefined), 25–30 per cent from healthy fat sources, and 10–15 per cent from protein – of which more later.

The energy balance equation

Whatever our body type, it's crucial that we understand the energy balance equation as this will significantly affect the way we shape up. To lose weight we need to create a negative energy balance – that is, consume fewer calories than those needed to maintain our current weight/energy output. If you want to gain weight and put on muscle, then you need to create a positive energy balance – which means consuming more calories than those required to sustain your weight and energy output. This will provide the necessary energy to build and maintain muscle. And to maintain weight, we need to match calorie consumption with calorie expenditure – creating a balanced energy balance.

(Note: The EPOC created by both weight and CV training will have a significant effect on energy balance – see page 54.)

Table 10 The energy balance equation			
kcal intake	**kcal output**	**Effect on weight**	**Energy balance**
1600	1600	none	balanced
2000	1600	increase	positive
1600	1900	decrease	negative

Note: 'Energy balance' refers to balance between calories consumed and calories expended.

Daily calorific requirements

If you look at food labels you'll see that most food products come with recommended daily allowance (RDAs) consumption guidelines – these are just that, and you should be extremely cautious of following them. Your body type, age, level of fitness and current diet will all have a very powerful influence on the number of calories you actually need to consume. For example, a mesomorphic rower or ecto-mesomorph desirous of weight (muscle) gain might need to consume 3000-plus calories a day in contrast to the recommended 2000 (or less) calories.

On page 24 you will find information on how to calculate your daily energy needs, while on page 25 you will find calorie burning figures for selected exercise types. To this, as indicated, you will need to figure in EPOC if you work out regularly 3–4 times a week (*see* page 54).

Training tip

In this increasingly technological age numerous gadgets are available to calculate metabolic rate and calorie expenditure.

Heart rate monitors
Many heart rate monitors have calorie counting functions. These use a calculation related to heart rate to estimate calories burned during exercise and everyday activity. These are, at most, 90 per cent effective (*see* page 49).

Metabolic rate measurement devices
These are worn on the upper arm and record metabolic rate by way of galvanic skin response. They are 100 per cent accurate. Originating from the medical world, they are now becoming increasingly available in the fitness market.

Macro-nutrients

Carbohydrate, fat and protein are macro-nutrients (vitamins and minerals are micro-nutrients, *see* page 119). Carbohydrate, fat and protein have very different bodily functions for general health, sports and fitness purposes. Table 11 identifies the energy release from macro-nutrients per gram (in calories). You'll see that fat contains about twice as many calories as carbohydrate and protein.

Table 11 Energy release from macro-nutrients (kcal)			
Macro-nutrient	Carbohydrate	Fat	Protein
Energy released kcal/gram	4	9	4

Carbohydrate (and fat) are the body's preferred energy sources during exercise. Although protein also supplies energy, this is usually only the result of prolonged CV workouts, when the body's stores of carbohydrate run low. This partly explains why ectomorphs or ecto-mesomorphs should be mindful of incorporating too much endurance training into their workouts if they want increased muscle size and strength, as the level of CV training could reduce their muscle protein stores and thus reduce muscle size.

CARBOHYDRATE

Carbohydrate should constitute 60 per cent of the daily diet. It is the body's prime fuel source when it is physically active. When digested, carbohydrate increases blood sugar levels and provides energy, through chemical reactions that occur in our muscles.

Carbohydrates are divided into simple types (sugars – also known as monosaccharides) and complex types (fibres and starches – also known as polysaccharides).

Simple carbohydrates contain one or two sugar units in their molecules, while complex carbohydrates contain from 10 units up to thousands of units.

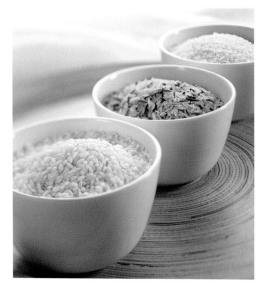

Glycogen – premium-grade muscle fuel

At rest, carbohydrate travels via the bloodstream to the liver and skeletal muscle where it is stored as glycogen (muscle fuel). Glycogen is a starch-like substance made up of numerous glucose molecules; it is used to fuel exercise. The amount of glycogen stored in the body is influenced by numerous factors, such as the amount of training you are doing, rest and carbohydrate consumption. It can only be stored in the body in limited amounts – around 375g. Glycogen needs to be replenished by carbohydrate consumption to maintain optimum physical capacity. In terms of energy potential, average glycogen stores amount to 1600–2000kcal – this would provide about enough energy for one day if we went without food.

Training tip

Begin your post-workout carbohydrate (glycogen) refuelling as soon as possible after your workout. Go for 1g of carbohydrate per kg body weight: thus if you weighed 60kg, you would need 60g of carbohydrate. You will capitalise on the fact that our bodies replenish their glycogen stores one and a half times more quickly in the two hours after a workout. Go for quick-releasing carbs (those with a high Glycaemic Index – *see* page 109).

Two large bananas or 1 litre of a 6 per cent carbohydrate isotonic sports drink will provide you with 50–60g of carbohydrate.

Glycaemic Index – the speed of energy release from carbohydrate

Many foods contain a mixture of simple and complex carbohydrates, so to measure their immediate energy release they are given a Glycaemic Index (GI) rating. This ranges from 1 to 100. Low GI foods release their energy more slowly compared to high GI foods. It is helpful to understand GI for everyday and specific fitness/sports nutrition purposes.

This is because it can help to control your blood sugar levels, thus maintaining your energy levels and avoiding over-eating. Table 12 identifies the GI of selected foods.

The smaller the size of food particles, the more quickly food is digested and the quicker it releases energy, hence the high GI of foods like bread and breakfast cereals.

Table 12 Selected carbohydrates and their GI

Type	GI value	Type	GI value
Sugars		**Fruit and vegetables**	
Glucose	100	Pineapple	66
Sucrose	65	Raisins	66
		Watermelon	72
Bread, rice and pasta		Banana	55
Bread – white	70	Orange	44
Bread – wholemeal	69	Plum	39
Pizza	60	Grapes	46
Rice – brown	76	Apples	38
Rice – white	87	Baked potato	85
		Chips	75
Breakfast cereals		Boiled potato	56
Cornflakes	84	Peas	48
Weetabix	69	Carrots	49
Muesli	56	Broad beans	79
Porridge with water	42		

Table 12 Selected carbohydrates and their GI (cont.)	
Type	**GI value**
Dairy products	
Ice cream	61
Custard	43
Full-fat milk	27
Skimmed milk	32
Pulses	
Red kidney beans	27
Butter beans	31
Soya beans	18
Biscuits and snacks	
Shortbread	64
Rice cakes	85
Tortillas	72
Muesli bar	61
Mars bar	68
Muffin	44
Peanuts	14

Factors to take into account when estimating the energy release of meals:

- Protein and fat reduce GI.
- For meals that combine two different GI-rated foods in roughly the same quantity, such as rice and kidney beans, total the GI of the two foods and divide by two.

- High GI foods should not be overly consumed throughout the day (apart from assisting training, as pre- or post-workout snacks, for example) because they release excessive amounts of the fat storage hormone insulin and create energy 'highs and lows'.

Training tip

Knowing the GI of foods will enable you to optimise food energy. For example, if you need a quick boost of energy before a workout, then a high GI food is a good choice. Low-GI foods eaten regularly throughout the day will provide you with a steady supply of energy, which will reduce (normally fat) cravings and help to control body weight.

Fibre

Fibre is important for our bodily functioning and is derived from plant sources. There are two types of fibre:

- Soluble fibre can be partially digested and may help to keep our cholesterol figures (see page 112) at healthy levels (good sources are beans, lentils and oats).
- Insoluble fibre cannot be digested; it therefore passes through the body and

helps the passage of other food through the gut. This food is also stodgy, fills us up, and can reduce over-eating (good sources are wholegrain bread and breakfast cereals, brown rice and fruit).

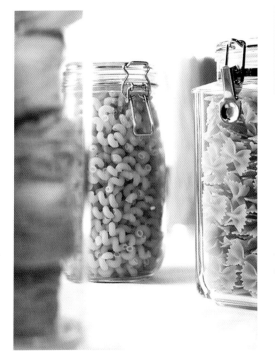

> ## Training tip
>
> Protein is just as important in the post-exercise refuelling process as carbohydrate. This is because it kick-starts muscle protein rebuilding. When weight training, muscle protein is broken down (a result of a metabolic process created by the muscles fibres involved being over-loaded and microscopic tears forming). This is a crucial consideration for all body types desirous of maintained or increased muscle mass.

Do you need to consume carbohydrate during your workouts?

I've added this comment here for serious trainers regardless of body type, and also to explain that you don't necessarily need sports drinks (containing carbs), despite what the manufacturers say. If you drink them when you don't really need to you'll simply add to your daily calorie consumption, which could lead to the addition of potentially unwanted weight.

If your workout lasts about an hour, then ingesting carbohydrate (through a sports drink or other source) will have little effect. Drinking water will be sufficient to maintain hydration. However, if you are a serious CV trainer working out for more than an hour, then carbohydrate can increase your exercise potential and slow down the emptying of your glycogen tank. You'll need to find out what food/drink strategy best suits you. As a guide, if you weigh 70kg you should consume 30–60g of carbohydrate per hour of exercise depending on workout duration; and if you weigh 60kg, this figure will be 25–50g.

Unrefined foods

Modern food processing and farming methods can reduce the vital vitamin and mineral content of foods below acceptable levels. In Table 13 you'll see why going organic and buying unrefined foods could optimise your mineral consumption. This will especially be the case once you have acknowledged what vitamins and minerals can do for your body.

Table 13 Food processing, mineral loss and selected foods			
Mineral	**White flour**	**Refined sugar**	**Rice**
Chromium	98%	95%	92%
Zinc	78%	88%	54%
Manganese	86%	89%	75%

FAT

Fat should constitute 25–30 per cent of our daily diet. It is an energy source for the body, but 1g provides more than twice the calories of carbohydrate and protein. As identified in Part 1 of this book, it can be stored on the body in various ways (e.g. as non-essential fat) to virtually infinite levels. It's this fat that is detrimental to health. Because certain body types can be more prone to certain diseases than others, it is vital to control fat consumption and to work out appropriately. For example, meso-endomorphs could profit from a CV-oriented programme to improve heart health, reduce hypertension and reduce body fat.

Fat serves crucial functions in the body; as well as providing energy, it is important for hormone metabolism, tissue structure and it cushions organs. A diet deficient in fat could lead to a lack of the fat soluble vitamins, A, D and E, and essential fatty acids.

Cholesterol and fat

Cholesterol is a part of all cell membranes. It is actually needed by our bodies as it contributes to the production of several hormones. Cholesterol is in part derived from the food we eat, but is in the main produced in the liver from saturated fats. Too much Low Density Lipoprotein (LDL) cholesterol is detrimental to (heart) health.

Although LDL cholesterol is commonly referred to as 'bad', it's only bad when its levels in the body are pushed up by factors that include a lack of exercise, obesity and excess consumption of saturated fats. LDL builds up in our arteries and restricts the passage of blood, leading to an increase in blood pressure. Unfortunately, it is not until there is 70 per cent arterial blockage that symptoms reveal themselves.

Ideal cholesterol levels are less than 5.7mmol/1 in the blood.

Very high cholesterol levels are more than 7.8mmol/1 in the blood.

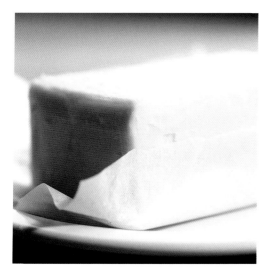

Different types of fat and suggested intakes

Saturated fat

Saturated fat should constitute less than 10 per cent of total fat consumption. Such fats are found mainly, but not exclusively, in dairy and animal products and are the most 'harmful'. In excess, they can raise LDL cholesterol and lead to heart disease. Examples are butter, cheese and the fat on meat – all are hard at room temperature.

Trans-fatty acids (TFAs) are particularly bad for health and result from the heating, refining and processing of saturated fats to prolong their shelf-life. TFAs are found in fast food. Some countries have started to ban or limit their use because of their potentially severe effects on health.

> ## Training tip
>
> Research indicates that ectomorphs are less likely to suffer from heart disease. This can in part be attributed to their lower levels of body fat.[vii]

[vii] *Folia Med (Plovdiv)*, 1996; 38(1): 17–21.

Unsaturated fats

- Monounsaturated fats are found in olive oil, nuts and seeds and can reduce LDL cholesterol and its negative effects. These fats are normally liquid at room temperature.
- Polyunsaturated fats are found in most vegetable oils, oily fish, nuts and seeds. They are liquid at room temperature and below. This type of fat can also reduce LDL cholesterol.

It's recommended that around 10 per cent of daily food consumption should come from these fats.

Essential fatty acids – omega-3 and omega-6 series

EFAs cannot be produced in the body and must be provided by food. They serve a crucial hormonal-like function as they can regulate numerous body functions. However, modern food processing methods can result in their nutritional value being significantly reduced.

Omega-3 EFA is found in some nuts and seeds, such as flax and pumpkin seeds, walnuts, soya beans and oily fish, such as sardines, mackerel, salmon, trout and herrings. Common omega-3 fatty acids include alpha linoleic-acid.

Omega-6 EFA can reduce LDL cholesterol. It is found in nuts, seeds, some vegetable oils (e.g. sunflower) and the germ of whole grains.

> ## Training tip
>
> **EFAs, and how they can assist your body type training**
>
> **Omega-3 EFAs:**
>
> - Improve oxygen and nutrient transport to cells.
> - Can reduce the risk of heart attacks.
> - Improve aerobic energy metabolism.
> - Help with strain injuries, as they have anti-inflammatory properties.
> - Benefit the immune system, thus reducing susceptibility to illness.
> - Can increase GH secretion as a consequence of sleep and/or exercise.
>
> **Omega-6 EFAs:**
>
> - Have anti-inflammatory properties.
> - Are good for the skin.

Recommendations as to the exact amount of EFAs that active people should consume often conflict. However, as a starting point, 9g of omega-6 and 6g of omega-3 per day should be aimed for.

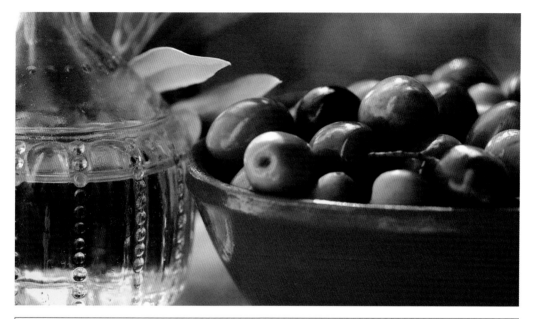

Table 14 The Essential Fatty Acids (EFAs) content of selected foods

Food	Omega-3 per 100g	Omega-6 per 100g
Salmon	3.2	0.7
Walnuts	3.0	3.2
Butter	1.2	1.8
Olive oil	0.6	7.9
Wheat germ	0.5	5.5
Olives	0	1.6

PROTEIN

Protein should constitute 10–15 per cent of our daily diet. Guys who are primarily training aerobically should aim for 1.6–1.8g of protein per kg; those aiming to add increased muscle mass should go for 1.8–2g. Protein is the building block of muscle.

Protein and amino acids

When protein is digested it's broken down into amino acids; some of these are called 'essential' (see Table 15) because they cannot be made in the body, while others are 'non-essential' because they *can* be made in the body, provided enough of the essential amino acids are present.

Table 15 Essential and non-essential amino acids	
Essential amino acids	**Non-essential amino acids**
Isoleucine Leucine Lysine Methionine Phenylalanine Threonine Tryptophan Valine	Alanine Arginine Asparagine Aspartic acid Cysteine Glutamic acid Glutamine Glycine Histidine (essential for babies only) Proline Serine Tyrosine

Table 16 Protein rating (biological value) of selected proteins	
Protein source	**Protein rating (biological value) out of 100**
Eggs	100
Fish	70
Milk	67
Brown rice	57
Peas	55

Protein can supply energy (4 kcal/g), but this is best avoided for all body types, as I have stressed throughout the book. This process occurs during very prolonged and intense periods of exercise when glycogen stores have been used up. Using protein as an energy source will reduce lean muscle mass.

What are the best proteins?

Proteins are given a rating out of 100 that indicates their level of inclusion of all the essential amino acids. This is termed biological value (BV). Proteins with the highest BV are best at being absorbed into the body and used for growth and repair (see Table 16).

Look out for whey proteins in supplements and food products as this is the most quickly absorbed of all proteins.

Turkey, cottage cheese, egg whites, soya beans, semi-skimmed milk and pulses are great low-fat sources of protein.

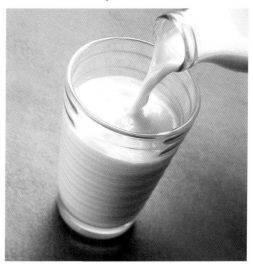

Table 17 How much protein do foods contain?

Food	Portion size	Protein (g)
Beef – fillet steak, grilled	105g	31
Chicken breast – grilled, no skin	130g	39
Poached cod	120g	25
Tinned tuna in brine – small can	100g	24
1 glass of skimmed milk	200ml	7
Eggs – size 2	1g	8
Cottage cheese – small carton	112g	15
Peanuts – roasted and salted (handful)	50g	10
Cashew nuts – roasted and salted (handful)	50g	10
Baked beans – small tin	205g	10
Kidney beans – 3 tbs	120g	10
Soya mince – 2 tbs	30g	13

Table 17 How much protein do foods contain? (cont.)

Food	Portion size	Protein (g)
Quorn mince – 4 tbs	110g	12
2 slices wholemeal bread	76g	6
Bowl of boiled pasta	230g	7

Adapted from Bean, A., *The Complete Guide to Sports Nutrition* (4th edition), page 21.

Soya, tofu and quinoa are rich sources of protein for both vegetarians and non-vegetarians. They combine high-protein content with little fat, and are also great carbohydrate sources. Quinoa can be obtained from health food shops and is a great rice substitute.

Training tip

Protein consumption prior to a workout could boost your muscle building as it primes the cells (in muscle fibres) for adaptation. For more information on protein and muscle gain, *see* page 130.

Micro-nutrients

Many guys are blissfully unaware of the positive effects the micro-nutrients can have on their bodies. Vitamins and minerals can seriously advance your training progress.

MINERALS
Twenty-two mainly metallic minerals make up 4 per cent of body mass; their main function is to balance and regulate our internal chemistry, for example, the maintenance of muscular contractions, the regulation of heart beat and nerve conduction.

VITAMINS
Vitamins are crucial in facilitating energy release from food, but do not produce energy themselves. There are two types:

- Fat soluble (e.g. A, D, E, K) – which are stored in the body.
- Water soluble, which cannot be stored in the body and derive from fruit and vegetables.

As with minerals, consuming excess amounts (above their recommended levels/reference nutrient intake – RNI) will not enhance their metabolic contribution.

Table 18 Selected vitamins and minerals and their fitness/sports and health benefits and reference nutrient intakes (RNI)

Vitamins/mineral	Function	Reference Nutrient Intake (RNI)	Selected sources
Biotin (B group vitamin)	Assists conversion of food into energy and glycogen manufacture and protein metabolism for muscle building	No UK RNI, 10–200ug/day is recommended	Egg yolk, nuts, oats and whole grains, dried mixed fruit
Calcium (mineral)	Assists muscle contraction, hormonal signalling, important for strong bones	1000mg/day	Dairy products, seafood, flour, vegetables, bread, pulses
Iron (mineral)	Can assist aerobic exercise, by promoting haemoglobin in oxygen-carrying red blood cells	8.7mg/day	Liver, red meat, pasta and cereals, green leafy vegetables, eggs, prunes, whole grains and dried fruit

Table 18 Selected vitamins and minerals and their fitness/sports and health benefits and reference nutrient intakes (RNI) (cont.)

Vitamins/mineral	Function	Reference Nutrient Intake (RNI)	Selected sources
Zinc (mineral)	Important for metabolising proteins, carbohydrates and fats	9.5mg/day	Lean meat and fish, eggs, wholegrain cereals, dairy products, wholemeal breads and cereals
Magnesium (mineral)	Boosts energy production and assists muscle contraction, plays a role in blood sugar stabilisation, which assists the balancing of energy levels. Aids the formation of new cells.	300mg/day	Green leafy vegetables, fruit, unrefined whole grains and wholegrain cereals, meat and dairy products
Copper (mineral)	Copper assists with collagen (soft tissue) formation and serves an antioxidant role. Encourages the production of red blood cells.	1.2mg/day	Beef liver, oysters, lamb, peanuts, baked beans, chick peas, wholemeal bread and wholegrain cereals

Vitamins/mineral	Function	Reference Nutrient Intake (RNI)	Selected sources
Table 18 Selected vitamins and minerals and their fitness/sports and health benefits and reference nutrient intakes (RNI) (cont.)			
C (vitamin)	Antioxidant. Assists cellular growth and repair. Aids absorption of iron from blood.	40mg	Fruit and vegetables, especially strawberries, oranges, tomatoes, green peppers, baked potatoes

ANTIOXIDANTS

Antioxidants include the vitamins A, C, E and beta-carotene and the mineral selenium. (Beta-carotene is what gives yellow and orange fruits their colour.) Once in the body it is converted to vitamin A and therefore performs the same functions – for example, helping vision in poor light. A diet rich in antioxidants can prevent cellular damage, reduce LDL cholesterol and defend the body against age-related diseases such as cancer and heart disease.

Antioxidants are especially important for all body types in hard training, particularly those involved in endurance activities. This is because intense periods of training can increase free radical cellular damage. To explain: oxygen fuels the heart and lungs and all bodily processes, including the energy release from

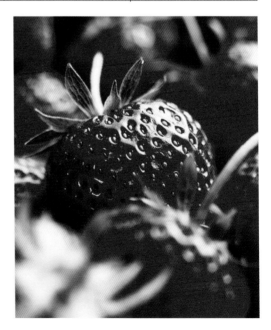

food. Unfortunately, oxygen metabolism can create unstable molecular fragments, which can damage cells if left unchecked. Antioxidant vitamins and minerals (and phytochemicals, which include bioflavonoids; both are contained in brightly coloured fruit and vegetables) can combat this cellular damage. (Note: Recent research has indicated that experienced trainers may suffer less from free-radical damage compared to those starting out on an exercise programme.)

Salt

You should restrict your salt consumption to 6g a day. Too great a consumption can increase

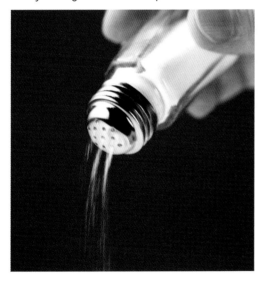

your risk of a heart attack. It's estimated that 85 per cent of UK men consume 9g of salt a day. To reduce salt consumption you need to consider the salt 'hidden' in ready meals and fast foods, as about 75 per cent of daily consumption comes from these sources, not from that added to meals already on the plate.

Diet or exercise?

Women (and an increasing number of men) turn to their diets before they consider exercise as a way of improving their health; and many go for 'fad' diets.

There has been a significant increase in these in recent years. Their merits are often debatable whatever their designers/advocates claim. It is beyond the scope of this book to go into the specifics of each, but some diets should be approached with caution. For example, low carbohydrate, high protein and high fat diets can have long-term health risks, such as heart and kidney damage.

Fluids

It is crucial, whatever your body type, that you keep hydrated for everyday health, fitness and sports training purposes. Around 75 per cent of the body is composed of water; keeping it hydrated, therefore, will optimise all bodily processes.

For everyday health, drink 2 litres of water a day. This can be derived from other drinks, such as tea (which is an antioxidant). For training or active days, go for 1 litre of water for every 1000 calories expended (*see* page 24 for how to calculate your calorific needs).

SPORTS DRINKS

As guys, we'll probably take note of what sports stars drink and promote, and sports drinks are often highly prominent. However, as I indicated on page 112, such drinks are not a necessity for CV workouts lasting less than 1 hour – where water will be sufficient for hydration needs. However, sports drinks can be of use for workouts in excess of an hour and as post-workout energy replacements for kick-starting protein re-synthesis and glycogen replenishment. Table 19 provides an explanation of the types of sports drinks currently available. Always read the label to check their contents.

ELECTROLYTES

Electrolytes are mineral salts (sodium, chloride and potassium, for example) that are present in bodily fluids. They regulate the fluid balance between different body compartments and the amount of fluid in the bloodstream. As an example, high cellular potassium levels increase the amount of water being pulled across a cell membrane, thus increasing the cell's water content. Sports drinks containing electrolytes have no direct effect on performance; however, sodium encourages the thirst mechanism (plain water or sports drinks without electrolytes will not do this). This will assist you to optimally hydrate.

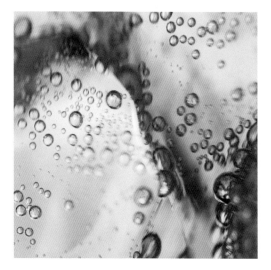

Advanced training tip

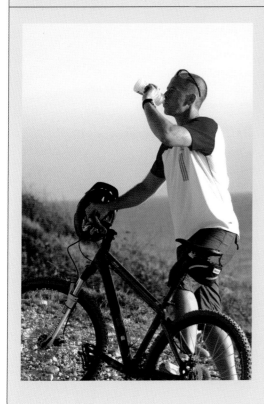

Weigh yourself before and after your workout. To calculate how much fluid you need, work on the basis that 1 litre of fluid is approximately equivalent to 1kg in weight. Lost a kg? Then make sure you keep topping up by 1 litre of water during your workout.

(Note: Take into account any clothes you may have discarded during your workout.)

Table 19 Different sports drinks

Type of sports drink	Constitution
Hypotonic (fluid replacement drink)	Contains lower particles of carbohydrate and electrolytes per 100ml than body fluid. An isotonic drink contains less than 4g carbohydrate/100ml, and this allows it to be absorbed faster than water. These drinks have a high osmolality.
Isotonic (fluid replacement drink/carbohydrate replacement)	Isotonic drinks have the same osmolality as body fluids, including water, and thus are absorbed at a similar rate (or faster) than water. Contain between 4 and 8g/100ml of carbohydrates.
Hypertonic (carbohydrate/energy replacement drink)	Hypertonic drinks have a higher osmolality than body fluids and are thus absorbed more slowly. Carbohydrate content: 8g/100ml. In the light of research indicating the importance of protein for recovery, a drink containing amino acids (protein) would also be highly beneficial. Minerals and vitamins contained in these drinks also stimulate carbohydrate and protein metabolism.

Ordinary drinks, such as fruit juices, are not suitable for use as sports drinks as they contain between 11g and 13g of carbohydrate and will not easily be absorbed into the body. Drunk in excess, they could also contribute to weight gain.

A loss of just 2 per cent in body weight (that's 1.5kg if you weigh 75kg) caused by dehydration could impair CV performance by 10–20 per cent.

Alcohol

To have a few beers or not have a few beers, that is the question . . . Well, alcohol is calorie dense and will not assist your training. Drinking in moderation is fine, but not in excess; at best it will lead to weight gain and, at worst, health problems.

A glass of red wine contains 85 calories, and a shot of vodka, whisky or gin each contain 55 calories. A unit is half a pint of standard strength (3–5% ABV = percentage alcohol by volume) beer, lager or cider, or a pub measure of spirit. A small glass of wine is about 2 units and an alcopop approximately 1.5 units (Food Standards Agency www.eatwell.gov.uk).

Men can drink up to 3 to 4 units of alcohol a day without a significant health risk.

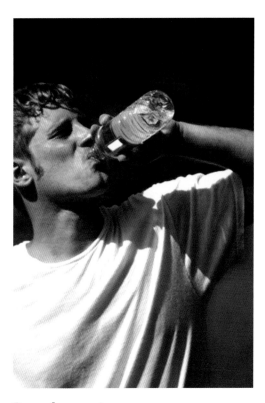

Supplements

Fitness and health supplements are big business. Men are particularly keen on using them and many gyms sell products on-site. But it's all too easy to believe the hype that goes with some of these. Although on many occasions a great deal of research goes into their production, not all of them may do what they say on the tub.

I have taken supplements on occasions in the past – notably creatine. However, I only did this after careful analysis of the product's claims. Being a fitness, sports and health writer perhaps made me more analytical. Also, as an international athlete I had to be careful for drug testing reasons as to what I took. In the following section you'll find a list of commonly used supplements together with an analysis of their claims.

Supplements can be beneficial and boost your body shaping, fitness and sports performance, but they should only be regarded as accessories to training. It is very important to realise just how important our food choices and calorific consumption is in terms of training and positively influencing body type. As indicated, micro-nutrients can have very significant positive effects on our body and its training response.

CREATINE

Creatine has been touted as the 'wonder' sports/fitness supplement and I must admit that most of its claims for improving strength and power and anaerobic performance have been vindicated by sports science. Creatine is produced naturally in the body from three amino acids. It is found in meat and fish, and is crucial for producing short-lived, but powerful, muscular energy.

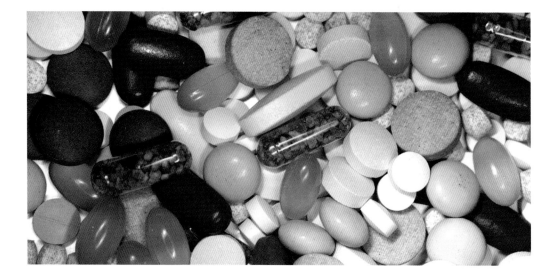

How does creatine supplementation work?

Basically, supplementing with creatine boosts your muscles' phosphocreatine (PC) stores, allowing you to train more intensely and with less 'fade'.

To benefit from creatine you need to take a loading dose, generally recommended to be 4 x 5g a day for 5 days and then a maintenance dose of 2g a day for a month. Once the month is up you will derive no further loading benefits and you should cease use for a further month, before starting the process again.

Body type and why you might want to use creatine

As indicated, the prime reason for taking creatine is to extend your anaerobic training capacity. With more fuel (PC) in your muscles you'll be able to train that bit harder. This can be beneficial for all body types. Here are some examples:

- Weight-training endomorphs, with their capacity for building larger muscles, will be able to achieve this more quickly, by performing a greater number of quality muscle-building repetitions.

- Ectomorphs will be able to combat their predisposition for reduced muscle mass by tackling tougher anaerobic workouts, and benefit from the associated 1-2.5kg gain in lean muscle mass that tends to occur just by taking creatine.

- Mesomorphs will be able to develop greater power and speed by performing successive sprints with less reduction in performance across reps, thus boosting their speed potential.

Are there any problems with using creatine?

Although the majority of research has found no adverse effects from using creatine, older people and those with kidney problems should consult with their doctors before starting a supplementation programme. Numerous research studies indicate that creatine can be beneficial for older populations in terms of increasing strength, muscle mass and functional mobility.[viii] Note also that the benefits of creatine for enhancing aerobic performance are virtually non-existent.

[viii] See, for example, *J Gerontol A Biol Sci Med Sci.*, 2003, Jan; 58(1): 11-19.

PROTEIN SUPPLEMENTS

Protein supplements have long been used by weight trainers and athletes. Protein is the key component in building, maintaining and repairing muscle. Weight training, for example, breaks down protein, and therefore optimum protein replacement (and optimum recovery) is needed to maintain and build bigger, stronger, more powerful muscles. As stated, you should aim for 1.8–2g of protein per kg of body weight if you want increased muscle mass.

Directions: Adults: One tablet daily, with food

Supplement Facts
Serving Size: One tablet

	Amount Per Serving	% Daily Value	
Vitamin A (14% as beta carotene)	3500 IU	70%	Niacin
			Vitamin B6
Vitamin C	90 mg	150%	Folic Acid
Vitamin D	400 IU	100%	Vitamin B12
Vitamin E	45 IU	150%	Biotin
Vitamin K	20 mcg	25%	Pantothenic Acid
Thiamin (B1)	1.2 mg	80%	Calcium
Riboflavin (B2)	1.7 mg	100%	Magnesium

CHILD RESISTANT CAP
SEALED for Y

Recent research has highlighted the importance of consuming protein prior to resistance and power training to prime muscle for positive adaptation. It has been well known for quite some time that supplementing post-exercise will increase the rate of protein synthesis and speed up the recovery and the growth of new, stronger muscle tissue.

Look for protein supplements containing whey as this is the most quickly absorbed of all proteins.

Note that too much protein (and too little carbohydrate) can lead to digestive problems, nausea, bad breath, osteoporosis and a lack of essential micro-nutrients being absorbed into the body.

Protein versus carbohydrate
When it comes to the 'protein versus carbohydrate diet/supplement' question, the answer is you need both. Carbohydrate is the body's key energy macro-nutrient. It's needed to keep your body's energy (glycogen) stores supplied and to fuel your training. Go for quick-releasing carbs (high GI) supplements, such as energy bars or drinks prior to and during workouts (particularly CV ones lasting in excess of an hour) and slower-releasing (low GI) meals and snacks throughout your day to keep your energy levels balanced, and to avoid cravings and fat accumulation (see Glycaemic Index, page 109).

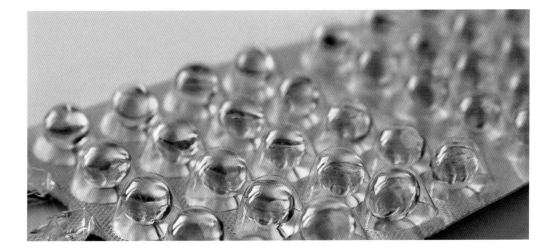

WEIGHT GAIN SUPPLEMENTS

Regardless of your body type, if you want to maximise your potential to build muscle then you will probably need to considerably increase your calorie consumption in order to provide both energy and sufficient muscle building materials (unless you are overweight, when a careful balancing act between calories in and calories out is required). This is because your 'normal' calorific consumption may be insufficient to do this (not enough calories consumed to exceed energy expenditure and thus promote muscle growth). In this instance, a weight gain supplement can be useful. This is because of the hundreds of additional calories it will supply. These supplements usually combine, quick-digesting whey protein with equally quick-energy-releasing carbs. Some also contain specific fats (essential fatty acids – *see* page 114), which are calorie dense, good energy suppliers and less likely to be turned into body fat.

Training tip

Supplements will only get you so far, and they should not be seen as substitutes for a carefully tailored, healthy diet, specific to your progressive training plan.

HMB (beta-hydroxy beta-methylbutyrate)

HMB is produced in the body from proteins containing the amino acid leucine. It's obtainable from a few foods, such as grapefruit and catfish. From a fitness and sports perspective, HMB has been shown to increase muscle size and strength and decrease body fat. HMB is believed to do this by inhibiting catabolic processes that would impair protein synthesis and muscle growth.[ix] HMB also seems to reduce muscular soreness created by training. The recommended dose is 3g per day.

Body type and why you might want to use HMB

As with creatine, you would use it to extend your anaerobic training capacity. (Note: Supplement manufacturers are producing 'all in one' products containing HMB and creatine (and other substances) in an attempt to maximise muscle growth and reduce muscular damage and aid recovery. Research indicates that combining the two supplements can result in strength gains, above that achieved if using one or the other.)[x]

GLUTAMINE

Glutamine is an amino acid found in muscle cells and is crucial for optimum immune system functioning. The commonly recommended dose is 2–3g per day (although with this supplement recommendations can vary greatly).

Glutamine should be taken immediately after exercise and again within two hours. However, research into glutamine's claimed benefits is at present much less consistent than for that produced for creatine, for example.

Note that if you are taking a protein supplement then you will invariably be increasing your body's glutamine stores in any case (look either for glutamine or glutamic acid as part of the product's contents).

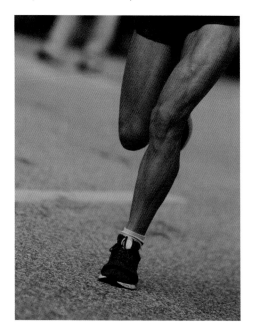

[ix] Sports Med, 2000, Aug; 30(2): 105–16.
[x] Nutrition, 2001, July–Aug; 17(7-8): 558–66.

Body type and why you might want to use glutamine

As it is claimed that glutamine can reduce muscular damage and maintain the immune system, it is worth considering its use for all body types in hard training. But I have to stress again that healthy, optimised eating can improve recovery after training and training adaptation and contribute significantly in maintaining general health.

FAT BURNERS

Fat burning products are designed to elevate the body's metabolic rate and mobilise fat as an energy source. Many contain the stimulants caffeine and guarana. Research has discovered the presence of International Olympic Committee (IOC) banned drugs such as ephedrine in some claimed 'natural' products. I therefore recommend that fat burning products should be avoided – regular training and a balanced diet will up your metabolic rate and burn fat naturally. As I've previously pointed out, regular training can elevate metabolic rate by as much as 20 per cent due to EPOC (see page 54). Note that regular eating is also crucial – the process of eating and digestion can account for 10 per cent of total daily calorie expenditure.

SUPPLEMENTS DESIGNED TO MAINTAIN YOUR BODY'S JOINTS

Recently there has been a growth in the promotion of joint-health supplements, often containing glucosamine sulphate or chondroitin. Taking these can be beneficial to all body types in training. These supplements need to be taken regularly as they serve an increasing protective function as levels build up in the body.

Glucosamine is a natural non-toxic compound found in the body. It is used in the manufacture of very large molecules found in joint cartilage; basically, these hold on to water, rather like a sponge, and in doing so provide cushioning for joints. A number of reputable surveys indicate that glucosamine can prevent knee joint (cartilage) narrowing (and the further development of arthritis) and reduce pain.[xi]

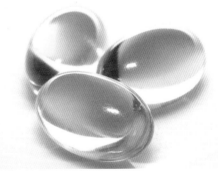

[xi] *Lancet*, 2001, 357: 251–6..

> ### Training tip
>
> You should always check the supplement product labelling and buy from a reputable supplier. Most products are designed for those with lactose intolerance. If in doubt about using a supplement, contact your doctor.

Chondroitin is another naturally occurring body compound. Like glucosamine, it is involved in the repair and maintenance of joints. Research is more limited at present, compared to that done on glucosamine, although those surveys that do exist indicate that it can reduce joint pain, increase mobility and reduce inflammation.

To build up working chondroitin and glucosamine levels in the body, try a combined supplement, ingesting 1500mg daily. The generally recommended ratio is 1000mg of glucosamine to 500mg of chondroitin.

As with other supplements, it is advisable to check with your doctor before taking glucosamine and chondroitin. For example, people with diabetes should check their blood sugar levels more frequently when taking glucosamine.

10 BASIC NUTRITION PROGRAMMES FOR SELECTED TRAINING GOALS AND BODY TYPES

It is beyond the scope of this book to provide detailed eating plans for various body types and training goals. I have therefore decided to focus on some common body type training goals, such as muscle gain and fat loss – as I have done in the practical training chapters. By studying their contents you will be able to pull out the key information that applies to you and construct a relevant dietary programme. Obviously you'll also need to follow the workout programmes provided in Part 2.

Goal: muscle gain

Many guys, regardless of body type, want bigger muscles – although those with endomorphic and mesomorphic tendencies will be at an advantage in achieving this goal. However, it is possible to increase muscle mass whatever your body type.

KEY WORKOUT TASK
Stimulate muscle growth via high-intensity medium/heavy weight training (CV work kept to a minimum).

KEY NUTRITION TASK
Ensure optimum protein consumption and timing to 'grow' bigger muscles. Ensure carbohydrate consumption maintains energy levels and replenishes glycogen levels. Consume healthy fat, to permit nutrient balance, but avoid unwanted fat accumulation.

DESIRED ENERGY BALANCE
Positive – up to 20 per cent more daily calories may be needed than those required to meet energy needs.

SELECTED BODY TYPE CONCERNS (WHERE APPLICABLE)
Ectomorphs. Of all body types, ectomorphs will have to ensure optimum nutrition to build more muscle, as their smaller muscle mass and higher metabolic rates can work against building muscle.

SELECTED BODY SHAPE CONCERNS (WHERE APPLICABLE)
Endomorphs. Being overweight. If you are overweight and want bigger muscles, then you are probably best suited to following a training programme that involves a high CV content initially to reduce body weight, before progressing to a more focused weight training programme. You will need to initially create a negative energy balance from your diet. You'll need to remove your 'fat' overcoat before tackling your muscles more directly. Once into your weight training phase, if you feel that you still want to reduce your weight further while building muscle, try this: reduce your calorie consumption by 15 per cent, 3–4 days a week on the days you don't train. On the days you *do* train, ensure that you create a positive energy balance of 10–15 per cent. You should avoid saturated fats (see page 107 for recommended macro-nutrient intake).

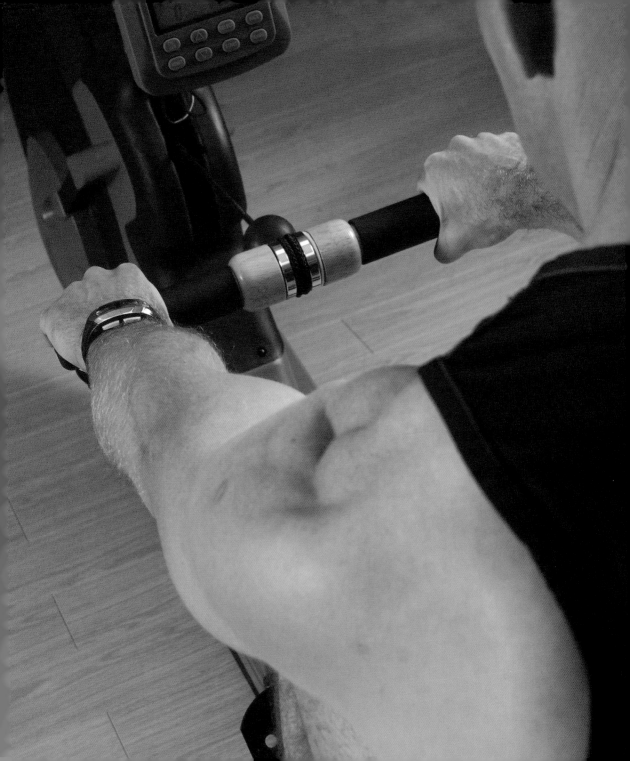

Training tip

Why does pre- and post-workout protein consumption optimise muscle growth?

Your workout will increase blood flow to your muscles, and with it numerous nutrients including amino acids (*see* page 116). Thus consuming protein 'around' your workout will ensure that the delivery and use of these amino acids is optimised within muscle cells for muscle growth.

Relevant pre- and post-workout fuelling will also create a positive hormonal response in your body by stimulating GH and testosterone release, which will boost your muscle building.[xii] Pre-workout, go for 20g protein. Post-workout, go for 20–40g protein over a 2-hour period.

The best protein bars will contain around 21g of whey protein (note they also contain carbohydrate and other products designed to refuel your body). Aim for 20–25g of protein with your meals.

[xii] *Int J Sport Nutr Exerc Metab*, 2004, June;
14(3): 255–71.

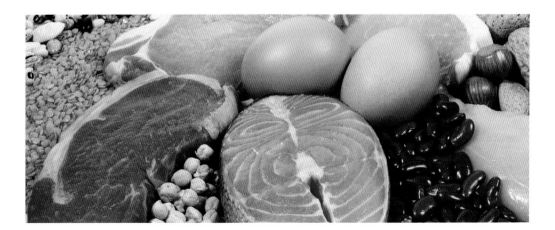

BUILDING MUSCLE AND CARBO-HYDRATE CONSUMPTION

Carbohydrate is crucial for a weight gain programme as it ensures that your body is optimally fuelled for exercise and everyday activity.

Note:
1) Eat too much carbohydrate and you could put on unwanted body fat once your glycogen stores have been restocked.
2) Eat too little carbohydrate and you run the risk of compromising your attempts to gain muscle as your body turns to its protein stores (your muscles) in an attempt to furnish itself with energy, and valuable muscle can be lost.

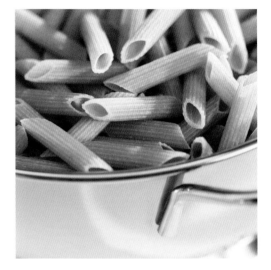

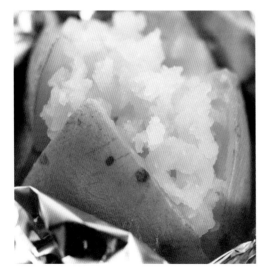

Calorie maths

If you weigh 80kg you'll burn around 17–18 calories per 0.5kg of body weight on a weight training day. To build muscle you'll need to create a positive energy balance. This would require 3200 calories.

Training tip

Ectomorphs could benefit from consuming denser (low GI) forms of carbohydrate, such as dried fruit and honey, due to their faster metabolisms. Endomorphs (and mesomorphs) prone to fat gains should go for natural fibre-rich carbohydrates, which are more filling.

It's recommended that you consume 5–7g of carbohydrate per kg of body weight per day. Ectomorphs or those with ectomorphic traits should consume carbohydrate towards the higher end of the range, and endomorphs and mesomorphs (and the overweight) towards the lower end. (Note: Both workout intensity and frequency can also have a significant effect on the amount of carbohydrate your body needs, as can EPOC (*see* page 54).)

Choose 'good' carbohydrates: potatoes, wholemeal bread, porridge, rice, pasta and fruit and unrefined sources where possible.

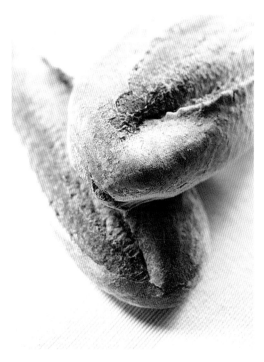

THE BENEFITS OF A LOW GI DIET FOR MAXIMISING MUSCLE GAINS

- Optimises glycogen replacement between workouts.
- Maintains energy levels.

Note that high GI foods should be used pre- and post-workout.

TIPS FOR PLANNING A LOW GI DIET

Balance your meals by including the following:

- Lean protein, such as chicken breast
- Fibre-rich carbohydrate
- Green vegetables.

Goal: fat/weight loss

With the growing obesity epidemic it is more than likely that the majority of men reading this book will be concerned with weight loss rather than weight gain.

KEY WORKOUT TASK

Emphasis on X-training – that's combining CV and resistance workouts to stimulate lean muscle mass, burn fat and increase everyday metabolic rate.

KEY NUTRITION TASK

As with increasing lean muscle, the training nutritional aim must be to ensure optimum protein consumption and timing to increase lean muscle mass. Carbohydrate consumption must maintain energy and replenish glycogen levels to optimise training readiness; however, it must be controlled to prevent a negative energy balance and weight gain. Healthy fat consumption is equally important – reduce total daily consumption to 25 per cent, increasing protein accordingly.

DESIRED ENERGY BALANCE

Negative. Use the guide on page 24 to work out your estimated calorific needs. Calorie reduction should be controlled and carefully implemented. You must avoid drastic cuts which could result in metabolic slow down. Try this: on non-training days, under-eat by 200–300 calories and maintain a balanced energy balance on your training days. After a while you may find that your lean muscle mass is declining (after shaping up). If this is the case, you will have to increase your calorific consumption to maintain your lean muscle – take a good look at your protein consumption. The best way to do this would be to create a positive energy balance on the days you train by 200–300 calories. On training days and non-training days you should maintain the same amount of protein consumption: 1.6–1.8g per kg of body weight. As a guide, an 80kg guy looking to lose weight would need 2500–2800 calories a day on non-training days.

BODY TYPE CONCERNS (WHERE APPLICABLE)

Mesomorphs and endomorphs are at greater risk of accumulating body fat, due to their tendency to have a slower metabolic rate.

BODY SHAPE CONCERNS (WHERE APPLICABLE)

Following on from the above, it is important to consider your actual body type as well as your body shape (*see* page 7) when you embark on a specific training and dietary programme designed for weight loss. To help, you might want to check out some photographs of yourself when yourself carried less weight so you can gauge your previous proportions. You

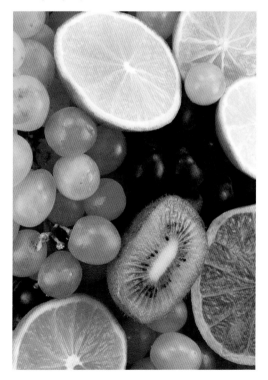

should also take into account your lifestyle then – to look at where you were perhaps burning more energy. You can then work out how you want to train to re-shape. This will also allow you to identify what type and how much training you will need to do to get the best results. As an example: if you were a dominant mesomorph before you gained weight, then your goal could be to train back to this type. You should note that your body type will respond to most types of training quickly and that you can be relatively free with food consumption when in training. However, the latter point will need to be mitigated by your current need to lose weight and the necessity of creating a negative energy balance and, of course, the need to still eat healthily.

WEIGHT LOSS TIPS

- Don't reduce your daily calorie consumption by more than 15 per cent. It might be tempting to cut back more significantly on calories, but doing this runs the risk of slowing metabolic rate as the body hangs on to the fewer calories it gets (this is sometimes known as 'famine/starvation mode'). Huge calorie cuts can reduce metabolic rate by as much as 45 per cent. Insufficient calorific consumption will also significantly impair our workout (and everyday activity) performance due to lack of body fuel.

- Create a negative energy balance. As there are 3500 calories in 0.45kg (1lb) of body weight, a 500-calorie daily deficit would theoretically get rid of this over a week. This negative balance can be achieved by calorie restriction and increased calorie expenditure through exercise. (Note: Your body type, age and genetic disposition will all affect your potential for weight loss.)
- Don't 'yo-yo' diet. Rapid increases and decreases in calorie consumption can throw the body's metabolism off-line and increase the risk of metabolic slow-down.

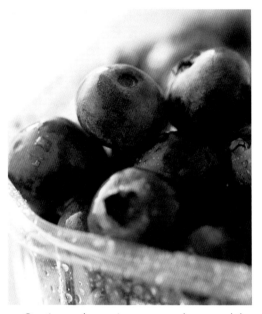

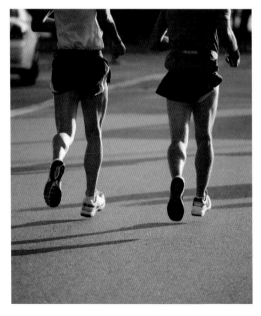

- Continuously monitor your workouts and the resulting increase in your fitness. As fitness improves, the body will become more exercise efficient. This means that you'll have to increase workout intensity to continue to burn as many or more calories than you did when you first started out. (Note: For safe training progression, do not increase intensity and duration at the same time.)
- Don't become preoccupied with where the calories you burn during your workouts come from (i.e. fat or carbohydrate). As I have indicated, what really matters is total exercise calorie burn.

- Don't believe that a specific 'fat burning zone' exists. All exercise options, both CV and resistance, can burn fat and help you achieve the body you desire (*see* page 52).
- Don't skip meals; calculate your calorific needs and eat frequently (five or six times) during the day. Research indicates that

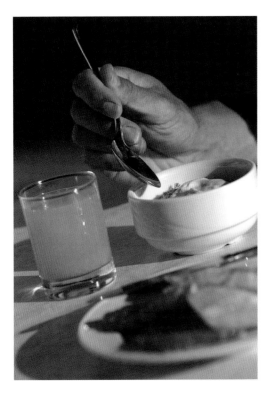

those who eat the most and train the most are usually the leanest and fittest.

SET-POINT THEORY

Sports scientists have argued that there's a control mechanism in our brain's hypothalamus that maintains a 'pre-determined' level of fat and weight for each of our bodies. That sounds good – and it is, until we put on weight over time and the body sets at a higher than previous level of weight (and fat). The good news is that research indicates that this mechanism can be challenged and returned to a lower set point, particularly by higher-intensity exercise, but not, apparently, by dieting alone.

What to actually eat!

I thought very hard about how I was going to get over to men the actual process of eating (I've provided a great deal of theory and what you should do). But what do you actually put on your table? In the end, I thought that providing the macro-nutrient content of selected healthy eating foods would be the best option (Table 20). You can then select those you like. You'll also see that the meals provided are simple to prepare!

Table 20 Macro-nutrient content of healthy foods				
Breakfast				
Food	**Kcal**	**Protein (g)**	**Carbohydrate (g)**	**Fat (g)**
1 cup (60g) porridge oats	241	7	44	5
300ml skimmed milk	99	10	15	0
1 tbs (30g) raisins	82	1	21	0
2 slices wholegrain toast	174	7	34	2
2 tsp olive oil spread	57	0	0	6
2 scrambled or poached eggs	160	14	0	12
3 Shredded Wheat	228	7	48	2
1 bowl muesli (60g)	220	6	40	5
4 heaped tsp honey	173	0	46	0
Glass of orange juice	72	1	18	0
1 tbs peanut butter	242	10	2	21
Low-fat fruit yoghurt (150g)	135	6	27	1
Egg large (raw)	74	6	Trace	5

Table 20 Macro-nutrient content of healthy foods (cont.)

Mid-morning snacks

Food	Kcal	Protein (g)	Carbohydrate (g)	Fat (g)
2 bananas	190	2	46	1
2 energy bars (66g)	309	7	40	15
2 apples	94	1	24	0
Peanut butter sandwich with 2 slices wholegrain bread and 1 tbs of peanut butter	174	7	34	2
	242	10	3	21

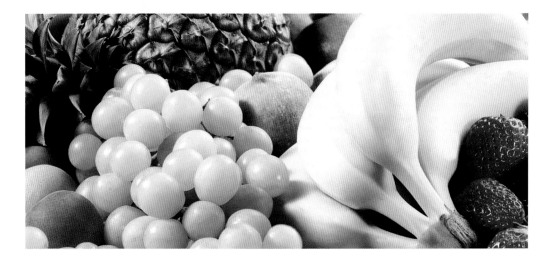

Table 20 Macro-nutrient content of healthy foods (cont.)

Lunch/dinner

Food	Kcal	Protein (g)	Carbohydrate (g)	Fat (g)
1 large baked potato (225g) with olive oil spread, tuna in brine (100g), salad (125g)	505	34	71	10
1 wholegrain pitta, 2 tbs olive oil spread, 2 slices turkey (70g), 1 bowl salad (125g)	343	25	36	12
Pasta salad, 2 tbs tuna in brine, large handful chopped peppers, 1 tbs olive oil dressing	563	33	82	14
Baked potato (as above), plus chicken (70g), sweetcorn (125g), salad (125g), 1 tbs olive oil dressing	373	35	106	15
Grilled turkey breast (100g), noodles (100g, uncooked), cauliflower	517	37	78	9

Food	Kcal	Protein (g)	Carbohydrate (g)	Fat (g)
Table 20 Macro-nutrient content of healthy foods (cont.)				
Large portion grilled chicken (120g), pasta (85g, uncooked), 1 tbs olive oil, large portion broccoli and carrots, pasta sauce	645	52	75	19
Grilled white fish (175g), large sweet potato, carrots, courgettes	549	45	90	3
Grilled salmon (175g), brown rice (115g), spinach	743	46	94	23
Sirloin steak grilled (90g)	206	30	0	9
Canned light tuna	116	26	0	1
Ham, extra lean sliced (90g)	131	20	1	5
Cod (90g)	105	23	0	1

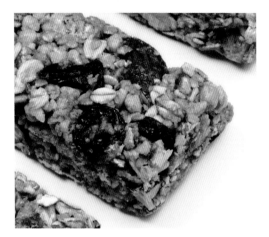
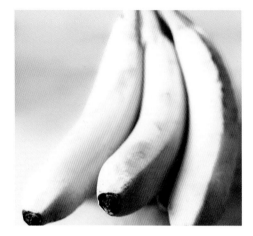

Table 20 Pre- and post-workout snacks				
Food	**Kcal**	**Protein (g)**	**Carbohydrate (g)**	**Fat (g)**
Protein bar/cereal bar (33g)	154	3	20	7
Meal replacement supplement (1 serving)	174	18	26	0
Orange	59	2	14	0
Low-fat yoghurt (150g)	135	6	27	1
2 bananas	190	2	46	1

Note: There are approximately twice as many calories in fat compared to protein and carbohydrate (approximately 9:4).

Source: Adapted from Bean, A., *The Complete Guide to Sports Nutrition* (4th edition).

Understanding food labels

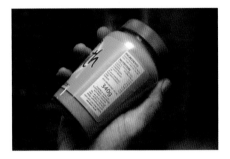

I tend to see food shopping as something to be done as quickly as possible – who wants to spend hours in the supermarket? However, spending just a little more time and getting to grips with food labels could make a huge difference to our body shaping, workouts and general health.

There is a legal requirement for the content of foods to be listed on packaging in the UK (this means that foods sold loose are currently exempt from labelling).

Key food labelling requirements:

- The content of the product must be clearly listed (many foods have names that are not relevant to the product).
- The content has to be clear to the user, but this might *still* not be clear unless you apply your grey matter! For example, 'fruit flavoured yoghurt' can contain artificial flavourings, while 'fruit yoghurt' must contain fruit.

- The food processing method used (if any) must be listed; for example, 'smoked salmon', 'roasted peanuts'.
- The weight (accurate to within a couple of grams) must be stated.
- Ingredients are then listed in order of weight – this must include water and any additives.
- Genetically modified foods must state this.
- Storage and preparation instructions must be provided.
- Energy value provided in kilojoules (kJ) and kilocalories (kcal).
- Macro-nutrient content (protein, carbohydrate and fat) listed in grams (g).
- The manufacturer may also choose to list the amounts of sugars, saturates, fibre and sodium.
- Information on other constituents, such as the type of fat in the product, can be listed. It is crucial to look for products that list all their ingredients. This will enable you to reduce those that are harmful to health (in large quantities, saturated and trans-fatty acids for example, *see* page 113).
- If the vitamin and mineral content of the product is listed as a percentage, then this is usually termed the Recommended Daily Allowance (RDA). RDAs are part of European Union legislation and represent an averaging of the RDA opinion from the EU member countries and their citizens.

GUIDELINE DAILY AMOUNTS

As noted, some products also provide guideline daily amounts. These give an estimate of the number of calories that men and women aged between 19 and 50 of 'normal weight and fitness' require. This figure is 2500kcal for men (and 2000kcal for women). These figures should, however, be viewed with caution as they don't account for specific body types and training status, for example.

Table 21 What's a portion (selected fruit and vegetables)?	
Fruit	
Apple, pear, banana, orange	1
Berries (strawberries, raspberries, blackberries, grapes	80g (1 cup full)
Melon, pineapple	Large slice
Tinned fruit (any type)	1/3 of a 400g tin
Fruit juice	Glass (150ml)
Dried fruit	1 tbsp
Vegetables	
Carrots/courgettes	1 large
Broccoli	2 spears
Mixed salad	Dessert bowl
Tomato	2
Cucumber	3 slices

Further advice on understanding units of food measurement

A gram is about the weight of a Smartie. Apart from calcium and potassium, the amounts of each nutrient required by the body each day are much less than a gram, so other, much smaller, units are used:

- The milligram – is abbreviated mg and is one-thousandth of a gram. There are 1000mg in a gram.
- The microgram – is abbreviated mcg and is one-millionth of a gram. There are 1000mcg in each milligram.

- The International Unit – is abbreviated IU. It is sometimes used instead of mg or mcg for some of the vitamins such as A, D and E where there is more than one form of a vitamin. IU express the biological activity that different forms of a vitamin exhibit.
- UK Reference Nutrient Intake – the daily amount deemed adequate to prevent deficiencies in 97.5 per cent of the UK population; this can also be displayed on food and is used by nutritionists.

CONCLUSION

Getting the most from your body type and changing your body shape for the better while improving your fitness is within your grasp. I've provided the information that will enable you to follow and devise the training and eating plans that will work for you and your goals – whether these are for weight loss, muscle gain or a more specific, perhaps sporting, goal. But before you shape up, reflect on the potential of your journey and think medium to long term when it comes to the time it will take to make lasting changes. Being a guy, I know we can be impetuous and want quick results, but you're not likely to get an action hero chest after a couple of weeks of training (no, *really*!). But you could after six months. Set short-term goals to push you on to your longer-term goals, and when you do reach your goal, set new ones and start the process again. Training and healthy eating will become a part of your life if you are consistent with your approach. But, having said that, don't obsess – a missed workout here and there is not a problem. It's the general, regular build-up of workouts under your belt that will reap dividends and (if relevant) reduce what's above it. Finally, enjoy yourself. Training should be (and is) fun. It's over to you from here on in.

INDEX